Poultry Health and
Management

Other books of interest

Animal Health
Second edition
David Sainsbury
0 632 03888 8

Primrose McConnell's The Agricultural Notebook
Nineteenth edition
Edited by Richard J. Soffe
0 632 03643 5

Dalton's Introduction to Practical Animal Breeding
Fourth edition
M.B. Willis
0 632 04947 2

Veterinary Epidemiology
Second edition
Michael Thrusfield
0 632 04851 4

Avian Medicine and Surgery
Second edition
B.H. Coles
0 632 03356 8

Poultry Health and Management

Chickens, Turkeys, Ducks, Geese and Quail

Fourth edition

David Sainsbury MA, BSc, PhD, MRCVS, FRSH, CBiol, FIBiol
1 Leys Road, Cambridge CB4 2AP

Emeritus Fellow of Wolfson College, University of Cambridge

Former Lecturer in Animal Health, Department of Clinical Veterinary Medicine, University of Cambridge

Blackwell Science

© 1980, 1984, 1992, 2000 by David Sainsbury
Blackwell Science Ltd
Editorial Offices:
Osney Mead, Oxford OX2 0EL
25 John Street, London WC1N 2BL
23 Ainslie Place, Edinburgh EH3 6AJ
350 Main Street, Malden
    MA 02148 5018, USA
54 University Street, Carlton
    Victoria 3053, Australia
10, rue Casimir Delavigne
    75006 Paris, France

Other Editorial Offices:

Blackwell Wissenschafts-Verlag GmbH
Kurfürstendamm 57
10707 Berlin, Germany

Blackwell Science KK
MG Kodenmacho Building
7-10 Kodenmacho Nihombashi
Chuo-ku, Tokyo 104, Japan

The right of the Author to be identified as the
Author of this Work has been asserted in
accordance with the Copyright, Designs and
Patents Act 1988.

First published by Granada Publishing 1980
Reprinted 1982
Second edition 1984
Reprinted by Blackwell Science 1987
Third edition 1992
Reprinted 1993, 1995
Fourth edition 2000

Set in 11/13pt Garamond and produced by
Gray Publishing, Tunbridge Wells, Kent
Printed and bound in Great Britain by
The Alden Press,
Oxford and Northampton

The Blackwell Science logo is a
trade mark of Blackwell Science Ltd,
registered at the United Kingdom
Trade Marks Registry

DISTRIBUTORS

Marston Book Services Ltd
PO Box 269
Abingdon
Oxon OX14 4YN
(*Orders*: Tel: 01235 465500
           Fax: 01235 465555)

USA
Blackwell Science, Inc.
Commerce Place
350 Main Street
Malden, MA 02148-5018
(*Orders*: Tel: 800 759 6102
                 781 388 8250
           Fax: 781 388 8255)

Canada
Login Brothers Book Company
324 Saulteaux Crescent
Winnipeg, Manitoba R3J 3T2
(*Orders*: Tel: 204 837-2987
           Fax: 204 837-3116)

Australia
Blackwell Science Pty Ltd
54 University Street
Carlton, Victoria 3053
(*Orders*: Tel: 03 9347 0300
           Fax: 03 9347 5001)

A catalogue record for this title is available from
the British Library

ISBN 0-632-05172-8

Library of Congress Cataloging-in-Publication
Data
Sainsbury, David
    Poultry health and management: chicken,
    turkey, ducks, geese, and quail/
    David Sainsbury. – 4th edn
        p. cm.
    Includes bibliographical references (p.   ) and
    index
    ISBN 0-632-05172-8
    1. Poultry. 2. Poultry–Health. I. Title
SF487.S15   1999   99-43235
636.5–dc21   CIP

For further information on
Blackwell Science, visit our website:
www.blackwell-science.com

Contents

Preface to First Edition

It appears as a surprising fact that, in spite of the enormous and exciting technical strides made in poultry husbandry and health in recent years there are remarkably few texts that bring the practical aspects of this together, so that all those concerned either with the keeping of poultry or who are eager to learn about it can find much that they require under one cover.

My own work brings me into close contact with poultry units and their problems, both in the UK and abroad, and I also have commitments in teaching both agricultural and veterinary students in the subjects of poultry management and health. This has convinced me of the need for a book that deals concisely with the application of our overall scientific knowledge to the practical management of poultry.

It may be helpful if I explain my approach to dealing with poultry management in this work. In the first place, I have explained briefly the overall structure of the industry and how it has tended to concentrate on a limited number of systems for each type of bird. It is also shown how great has been the increase in efficiency in recent years with the poultry industry very much in the vanguard of all agricultural developments. Following this introductory section, which includes an explanation of the breeding policies of the hybrid poultry companies, there are explanations of the nutritional needs of all classes of poultry.

The importance of poultry feeding cannot be over-emphasised, and I hope that this has been dealt with sufficiently, as a knowledge of this is fundamental to good management. So also is a complete understanding of the environmental needs of poultry and the ways in which these may be achieved in a practical manner. Thus, I deal in these sections with the air temperature, lighting and ventilation needs of poultry, together with the construction and thermal insulation of the poultry house. These are all items of management which are very much under the control of the poultryman himself and these sections have been written to give him the underlying knowledge to deal with these aspects.

In the chapter on 'Disease and Intensification', my philosophy is explained in that every effort must be concentrated into the prevention of disease, and with a good understanding of the factors that cause disease, healthy poultry are a practical reality!

The subject of poultry health forms a major part of this book; so far as possible I have attempted to avoid the 'dictionary of disease' or 'pathological' approach, which is much more for the specialist.

I have explained the principal systems of poultry management and even those currently less popular, since there is plenty of evidence that most systems of management have a part to play somewhere in the world. Poultry husbandry has become a highly international matter; for example, broiler chickens are reared in almost precisely the same way in the USA as in the UK, or in Africa, Asia or the Middle East. This is meant to be a book for international use, which can enable the poultry keeper to obtain pleasure and profit from rearing productive and healthy stock. Vast waste takes place throughout the world due to the inefficient use of our resources and it is our duty to make certain that when poultry are kept, their great potential productivity is thoroughly ensured by their correct management.

Fairly brief sections have been given on the husbandry of turkeys and ducks, emphasising in particular those aspects that are different from the domestic fowl. The consideration given in the earlier chapters is not, however, exclusive to the chicken but bears in mind the need of other poultry.

I am not ashamed to admit that I have found my involvement with all aspects of poultry keeping over a period of 40 years – in fact, since I kept laying birds semi-intensively and fattening chicken in individual pens 'Sussex style' from the age of ten –to have been an enormously pleasurable one. It does not matter how big or small a unit is, the birds still respond acutely to their management, and if I can instill some of this enjoyment and attitude into the reader, a great deal of the aim of this book will have been achieved. Bibliographies of further reading are given where a deeper understanding can be obtained and I hope the books quoted will be sought out.

Preface to Fourth Edition

This is the fourth edition in the 20 years since this book first appeared and every time a new edition has been produced it has been necessary to make significant amendments. The third edition had extra sections on quail and geese and those alternative systems of husbandry which reduce the intensity of housing and management. Readers were also introduced into the great 'food scares' saga, which appears to be destined to run and run. Since then there have been considerable advances in nutrition, housing and management, in health control and now into the production of organic poultry products. All these topics are dealt with and it will be quite apparent that the technical enhancement of poultry production continues apace, with certain very profound changes emerging.

David Sainsbury

Acknowledgements

The greatest pleasure in the production of this book is to express thanks to all those who have given help. James Hunnable, John Baron and Janey Barnard of the Cobb Breeding Company provided important information and illustrations, Arnold Elson, who is an expert consultant on poultry housing, equipment and systems, has granted me permission to reproduce information and diagrams on alternative and other management systems. His work is especially applauded, together with that of his colleagues in the Agricultural Development and Advisory Service to whom the whole industry is grateful.

My thanks are likewise extended to Mr G.E.S. Robbins for allowing the use of diagrams and material from his books on quail. He is an undoubted expert on the subject, and his books are listed in the section on 'Further Reading'. Tables 4.1, 4.2 and 4.3 are reproduced by kind permission of the Ministry of Agriculture, Fisheries and Food and Table 11.2 by permission of Merck and Company, Rahway, New Jersey. I also thank Mrs Wyeld for permission to use the tables on rations for ducks. The poultry industry is also served with great distinction by John Farrant, MBE, Editor of *Poultry World*, and his colleagues and Terry Evans and David Martin, Editor and Technical Editor, respectively, of *Poultry International*.

My further thanks go to Richard Phillips of Breckland International, who pioneered the Pecka-Block and Ron Parry of Maywick International, who has contributed so much to the brooding and heating of poultry housing. They have supplied some excellent illustrations.

My further thanks go to Thomas E. Whittle, who gave wonderful service to the poultry industry for many years at the Poultry Science Department at Auchincruive, Ayr and recently produced the splendid work, *A Triumph of Science*; also to Colin Rushmere and Peter Williams of Vernagene at Bolton, Geoffrey Cartwright of Orffa Ltd at Congleton, David Thacker and Matthew Ward of Crown Chicken, Kenninghall, David Peters of Intervet, Ronald Freeman of Anglian Farm Supplies, Clive Gerdler and Richard Skoyles of Vericore of Preston.

Finally, my grateful thanks to Richard Miles and colleagues at the publishers, Blackwell Science, and to my secretary Joy Tuck, who have given invaluable and constant support at every stage of the book.

1 Poultry – Their Health and Management: Introduction

The background

In a span of some 50 years there have probably been greater changes in the methods of keeping poultry than in any other sector of the world's livestock agricultural production. It has now become the most intensive of all branches of livestock farming. In many countries poultry are now ahead of all other livestock in economic importance. Table 1.1 shows how remarkably productivity has improved and systems of management have changed within the past 40 years. In 1960 all systems for the production of eggs recorded an average number of eggs per annum of 185 per bird. In 1999 it was not far off 300 and indeed in cages it was over 300. Also, whereas in 1960 there were over 30 per cent on free range but only 19 per cent in cages, in 1999 the figure was 15 per cent on free range and 80 per cent in cages.

Table 1.1a Yield per laying fowl (eggs per annum – September to August)

Systems of management	1960–61	1971–72	1976–77	1989–90	1997–98
Free range	166	190	192	220	276
Battery cages	206	235	245	290	311
Deep litter and barn	187	209	224	250	287
All systems	185	230	243	253	294

Table 1.1b Percentage distribution of laying fowl by systems of management

Systems of management	1960–61	1972–73	1979–84	1988–92	1998–99
Free range	30.9	4.5	1.9	13	15.5
Battery cages	19.3	88.1	96.1	85	80.1
Deep litter and barn	49.8	7.4	2.0	2.0	4.4

These figures are certain to show rapid changes, with a strong trend away from cage systems due to the pressure from welfare interests, helped along by legislation. Indeed, European legislation is threatening to outlaw all cage systems for poultry by the year 2013 within the European Union.

Table poultry are produced very largely intensively, although there is also a growing market for free-range birds that are reared with access to pasture. Productivity improvements in table poultry have been remarkable. In 1952 it took some 13 weeks to produce a 2.0 kg bird consuming 6.0 kg of food; in 1999 a 2.0 kg bird was grown in approximately 6 weeks at a consumption of 3.6 kg of food.

Intensification

Poultry have undoubtedly led the field in the advanced technical process required for intensification; indeed, the lessons learned by the poultry keeper have often been copied by those rearing other livestock. It is true to say that any up-to-date guide to poultry health and management can be consulted with advantage by all those who keep any farm livestock, as much of the technology, if not the husbandry, is common to all, with poultry usually the progress leader.

There are a number of well-defined reasons why poultry keeping became such an intensive operation. It is appropriate to consider the problems of keeping birds outdoors. Food costs become much heavier because colder conditions often require a large percentage of the food merely to keep the birds warm and to provide the energy required for exercise. There may also be losses of food when it is gathered by wild birds, rodents and other predators, while labour requirements are infinitely more demanding and much greater areas of land are required. These disadvantages represent the main reasons why the poultry industry went intensive in the 1940s and 1950s, but since that time there have been further powerful arguments for the development of much better environmental control in poultry houses. First, for reasons of improved productivity, the need to control lighting in duration, frequency and intensity made it highly desirable not only to house poultry, but also to keep them under artificial light programmes in windowless houses. Later on, investigations on the physiological needs of poultry showed the importance of warmer housing as a means of improving productivity and lowering feed costs, while the need to fully *control* the feeding with many types of poultry, rather than just to provide the food, has further emphasised the desirability of controlling the total environment of birds of all ages. Finally, keeping the birds under control has enabled better disease prevention and the effective administration

Plate 3 Broiler breeders in a hot climate in naturally ventilated houses but with electric circulating fans mounted under the ridge.

Plate 4 Hatching eggs being placed in the sanitising machine before entry to the incubator.

left world-wide. While the responsibility they bear is immense, there is every indication that they can meet the need, and the fears sometimes expressed that the genetic pools are becoming too concentrated do not stand up to practical scrutiny.

The fact is that each company maintains an enormous supply of breeding material in its own right, and the skills are available to make use of it. It is an intriguing fact that the majority of the large breeding companies are in the hands of industrial conglomerates. Of these, food and pharmaceutical concerns have predominated, although in more recent times several have sold to the management in the realisation that the job is best left to those who understand it.

2 Health, Disease and Intensification

In the planning of modern intensive poultry units very little attention has been given to the effect of such intensification on disease and its incidence. This is equally important for fully housed poultry or for modem 'free-range' systems. Yet there is now abundant evidence that the productivity of poultry may fall as the size of the unit increases and when there is no apparent difference in management between sites. In a survey carried out by the author, broilers showed a variation in finishing weight at the same age from 2.1 kg in groups of 20 to 1.4 kg in groups of 30 000, with an almost *pro rata* relationship with groups of between 50, 100, 500 and 10 000. These differences occurred with birds from the same genetic material, eating similar food and without any obvious disease. A similar trend was shown in a survey carried out by the Agricultural Development and Advisory Service, which showed that broiler growers with a location size of between 595 and 738 m^2 – a modest range – gave the best performance, which is highly significant. Then for each doubling of location size beyond this average, weights decreased by 0.09 kg. The decline in weight was almost certainly due to the increased incidence of disease, and good use should be made of such accurate figures by the poultry industry to modify old units or plan new ones. The same experience has been shown with productivity in laying units – above a certain size productivity tends to fall away, although the magnitude of this is less in mature birds than in the young or growing bird. This is because in the former case immunities to disease tend to be established, while in the grower they are often either absent or insufficient to resist a challenge.

The apparently greater disease incidence in the larger unit is not necessarily due to obvious 'clinical infections' and the nature of the problems goes undetected. It is interesting that it has been reported that some animals can produce substances that inhibit the growth of smaller animals of the same species. The result is that the more rapidly growing animals survive at the expense of the slower growing ones. This phenomenon could be a factor in the depression of overall weight in large groups and the increasingly uneven growths that occur, in addition to the problems of disease and behavioural stress.

Husbandry size and efficiency

In relation to the facts given in the preceding section, it is one of the encouraging elements in poultry husbandry that, in spite of mass production methods and increasing reliance on automation, birds are still highly responsive to the effects of management. No more and no less than other farm livestock, birds with the same apparent housing and nutrition facilities and of the same genetic material are still capable of giving vastly different results, depending on the care taken with management. It is significant that the farms which head the tables of productivity are usually the smaller units under the personal supervision of the owner. These are more efficient as a way of producing *any* poultry products, on several grounds.

If productivity is better and food conversion improved then clearly the world's resources are being used more economically. Thus, the very large units may seem profitable as a purely financial exercise because of the very large amounts of stock. However, as a means of utilising the world's limited resources this may not be so at all and if productivity, food conversion and mortality are worse and disease incidence is higher, then it could be a bad bargain and may also produce an inferior end product. With a smaller unit, it is also easier, and more likely, that better use will be made of the 'waste products' such as manure and litter, because it can be used on the land nearby, keeping storage and handling to a minimum. In future, if this pressure on the need for economy grows as it should, then the highly efficient units must not be so large as to be incapable of giving the best biological results and unable to dispose of their waste products easily and usefully.

'All-in, all-out' poultry management

Soon after poultry farming entered the era of intensive management it was established that there were considerable advantages in following what is termed an 'all-in, all-out' programme. This means that all the birds in a unit are housed at the same period, this period being as 'tight' as possible. They are then taken through to the end of the growing or productive period so that the whole unit or site can be cleared of livestock and of all muck, both within and without the houses, and then subsequently disinfected, fumigated and rested for at least a couple of days. Such a process has an enormous amount to commend it and the list of advantages given below is impressive. It may be pertinent to mention that in very recent times it has become less common to insist on the 'all-in, all-out' procedure and to rely rather more on vaccines, antibiotic and chemotherapeutic medicines as a means of controlling disease. All such means have a part to play, but it is very doubtful whether a system can survive at all if it is utterly dependent on them, especially as the availability of licensed medicines is diminishing and the public concern about residues of additives in poultry products is growing. The advantages of an 'all-in, all-out' policy are listed below.

- The clearing of all living animals off the site can be the biggest factor in eliminating most, if not all, organisms capable of causing disease. The more frequently this 'depopulation' is practised, the more likely it is that any build-up of disease will be prevented.
- Once the site has been completely cleared of birds it is possible to apply the most robust and effective programme of disinfection and fumigation, so progressing towards an elimination of bacterial, viral, fungal and parasitic infections.
- The maintenance of birds on a site within a close age range makes for a more uniform state of immunity to disease. Mixed ages lead to an immunological confusion, so that the uptake of vaccines or treatments is less satisfactory. It is certainly much more difficult for the correct administration of disease prevention programmes, as some birds will almost certainly not respond, or will receive the treatment at the wrong time.
- There are sound and practical husbandry advantages. If a site is filled at one time there is only one unavoidable disturbance. Nothing more will be altered, until the site is cleared. If units have birds coming and going at irregular intervals, the disturbance occurs at various times and can lead to hazards on health and behavioural grounds.
- It may also be considered an advantage if the operator can have a pause in the exacting task of management. Maintenance of equipment can also be properly carried out between batches so that there are likely to be far fewer breakdowns.
- In recent years, with the great increase in intensification, there have been serious problems around poultry sites that are in continuous use of nuisance caused by flies breeding in the manure and other organic matter. Large sites often have poor arrangements for muck disposal. Smells can cause highly objectionable conditions for nearby residents. An 'all-in, all-out' site can limit the feasible size of a unit, which is not a bad point in itself, but above all can make it much more practicable to eliminate breeding areas for insects and rodents.

It may be emphasised that the merits of depopulation are in inverse proportion to the age of the birds; it is less important with the adult because by the time a bird has reached maturity it may have achieved a satisfactory immunity to disease.

Environmental control and health

Probably the first group of diseases that come to mind when considering the relationship between environment and disease is the respiratory complex. It is inevitable that under intensive conditions the likelihood of birds being infected with respiratory ailments is greater than those kept extensively or semi-intensively. Environmental control has certain major functions. First, it must provide ventilation arrangements that constantly bring in fresh air and draw off stale air, gases and other pollutants. In this way, respiratory by-products that may contain disease-producing organisms will be removed. It must, however, perform this vital function in such a way that a uniform movement of the air is applied to the whole area inhabited by the birds, so exchanging the old air with the new in a manner that is virtually imperceptible to the stock.

In Chapter 7, details are given of the practical way in which good ventilation can be achieved, but the reasoning behind the systems should be understood.

As birds are placed in greater concentrations, it becomes increasingly difficult to get uniform air movement. Far too little attention is given to this and relatively too much to the capacity of the fans, important though the latter may be. It is clear that birds housed intensively do react quite markedly to comparatively minor variations in temperature and air movement. Several studies on the performance of birds in cages have shown that there is a significant difference in various locations, with particular emphasis on the deleterious effects of cold and draughts. At the other end of the scale, the author has frequently been distressed by heavy mortality occurring in mechanically ventilated poultry houses after sudden rises in the ambient temperature and humidity. To some extent, these may have been due to higher stocking densities, but more frequently they seem to have arisen from poor siting and design of the fresh air inlets. Mortality has also occurred when the fan capacity has been even more than adequate.

Birds' reaction to illness

When birds become ill with elevated body temperatures and reduced appetites and water consumption, they tend to feel the cold more, just as the human subject does when sick. They will then try to move together, huddling in areas of low air movement. Just how much this aggravates the problem it is impossible to say precisely, but it can be surmised that the build-up and intensification of the disease-producing organisms is inevitable under these circumstances, causing a vicious circle of yet more disease challenge to the birds. In accommodation where heat is available, one practical procedure is to increase the heat input when the birds are ailing to raise the temperature by several degrees. This not only tends to persuade the birds to separate from one another but also ensures that the ventilation rate is not merely maintained but is increased to support any treatment being used. In emphasising the importance of keeping warmth up to counteract infection, it is also pertinent to stress that many viruses have optimal multiplication temperatures a degree or two below the normal body temperature of the host so that chilling will promote the harmful effects of these pathogenic organisms.

Control of air movement

It has been stressed that a uniform diffusion of the air across the house is essential at all times. There are two quite different ways of achieving this. The most common is to introduce the air into the building at a low speed and either deflect it away with a baffle or diffuse it through slats, perforated inner linings such as slatted hardboard or media such as mineral wool, glass wool or canvas. These are frequently used to advantage in 'rescue operations' to diffuse the air into houses with badly designed inlets, or to reduce the unfavourable effects of high winds, but there is a danger that they may reduce the total air entry by restricting the efficiency of fans. Also, if they are neglected they may become clogged with dust and lead to a build-up of infection. They thus require expert installation and use, and are considered fully in Chapter 7.

The second approach is to bring the air in at a high velocity and either to deflect it abruptly against a baffle board close to the inlet or to direct the air well away from, and usually above the birds, so that the draught potential has quite disappeared by the time the air reaches the birds. It is impossible to state categorically which is the best system; indeed, from results in the field it seems that each system, properly designed, can produce equally favourable results. Each form of house seems to have a system most appropriate to its design, and use should be made of the right one in assisting the maintenance of the health of the birds. So many houses have a mixture of different systems that no logical pattern can be said to exist and the essential point to grasp is that most failures occur because they are ill-conceived mixtures of systems.

Another major practical factor in maintaining uniform conditions is the way in which the fans are controlled; there is no need for birds to be subjected to the stress of badly controlled fans. Fans with speed controls enable gentle changes to be made in fan speeds as the climatic conditions change.

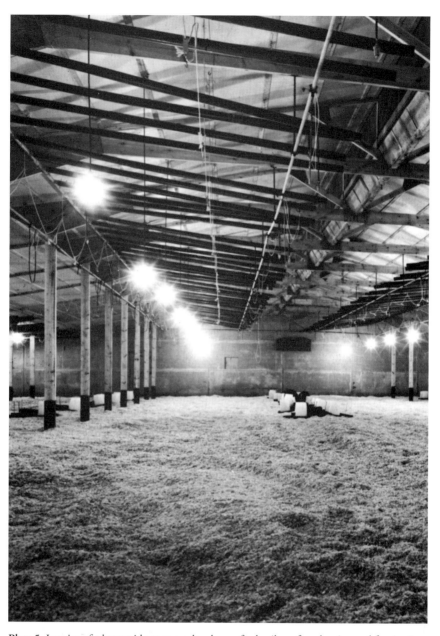

Plate 5 Interior of a large wide-span poultry house for broilers after cleaning and fumigation. Note the litter on the floor, which is usually put in place between disinfection and fumigation procedures so that it can benefit from the formaldehyde gassing. The automatic feeding vertical piping is seen under the ceiling where it is safely placed during disinfection and fumigation. Ventilation is by side-wall fans and controllable ridge intake – a satisfactory system using high-speed air flow at roof level.

Most modern arrangements have regulating systems that *gradually* change the speeds of the fans and a variable minimum rate can be changed as required, according to the age and the stocking rate of the birds. The arrangement is economic where there are large houses requiring a number of fans but a less sophisticated arrangement may be used satisfactorily with a speed regulator reducing the fan speed to 10 per cent of the maximum. In small houses, a unit of two fans for example, one thermostatically controlled and the other on manual regulation is as good as the most sophisticated systems. Indeed, it may have certain advantages because it leaves some important functions to the stockman and does not leave everything to an unfeeling automatic thermostat or thermistor. Recently, this type of approach has been more positively advised in multi-fan systems since it requires very simple equipment with little chance of error. In large installations speed regulation can be avoided by bringing in fans in series at top speed. This is a less complicated system and is cheaper to install, run and maintain.

In widespread experience there have been clear indications of the striking advantages of maintaining laying birds in a warm environment of not less than 21°C (70°F) or more than about 30°C (86°F) with relative humidity between 50 and 60 per cent. If such high temperatures are to be maintained in laying houses all the year round – and in any case they are essential during the early rearing stages of chicks – it places an increased emphasis on the importance of maintaining uniform and constant ventilation and the very highest standard of thermal insulation. Such high temperatures require especial care in housing and all the ventilation must be under impeccable control.

Brooding

The detailed practicalities of this will be dealt with in an ensuing chapter but it is pertinent to mention some of the vital features with respect to health. A great deal of work has been done on methods of brooding, or methods and techniques providing warmth in the early days of life. Over some years of work at Cambridge it was found that the best results were obtained from heating systems that combined radiant and convected heat. In practical terms, this means an arrangement that provides a warm area for resting birds and a slightly cooler area for movement. However, since birds brooded on the floor must be encouraged to use as much of the floor area as possible right from the beginning, the movement area must still be evenly warmed and an absolute minimum temperature of 21°C (70°F) is advised. In practice, to ensure that the temperature never drops below this, it is much better to specify a minimum somewhat higher than this, say 24°C (75°F). Also it is essential that the chicks can be readily inspected and there is a good uninterrupted air circulation all round them. For these reasons, brooders of largely radiant heat output are favoured, that can be placed well above the birds. The rather heavy insulated canopied type, close to the floor, is no longer necessary in modern buildings that are well insulated overall, and they also have the disadvantage that they concentrate the chicks in too limited an area and make proper inspection much more difficult.

An alternative arrangement that has gained increasing popularity, is the use of one or more hot air blower heaters that raise the whole house temperature to the 'required level'. However, the determination of the 'required level' raises some problems. On the one hand, if health and appetite are to be ensured, the temperature must not be too high, but as opposed to this, hot air requires an essential velocity to distribute the heat, so that the cooling effect on the bird is greater than with a radiant brooder. In this connection there are two essentials. First, there must be an arrangement to duct the air, or so deflect it in such a way that it does not have to be blown long distances creating draughts, dust and regions of the environment unacceptable to the birds. Second, while the initial temperature must be high – about 31°C (88°F) – the method of compensating for the disadvantage for an overall high figure is to reduce this as soon and as regularly as possible. For example, if the temperature starts at 31°C (88°F) and is reduced by 0.6°C (1°F) daily, it will promote the qualities required in the birds. An additional problem with whole house heating is the effect on humidity. With a high temperature over the whole house, the relative humidity will be very low – 30–40 per cent. It is known, however, that a higher relative humidity, up to about 60 per cent, is better for the chicks. Higher humidity promotes good feathering and growth and provides the best environment to enable the birds to resist the effects of any respiratory infection. In moister atmospheres the organisms causing respiratory challenge will generally perish more quickly and the mucous membranes that line the respiratory passages of the birds will remain in a healthier state. Nevertheless, it appears that at both *very high* and *very low* humidity, air borne organisms that can cause disease are likely to remain viable for longer periods than where the humidity is in an intermediate range. High humidity near saturation, such as is found in the winter months, is especially favourable to the survival of respiratory organisms and this may be one of the factors contributing to the much higher incidence of respiratory disease in cold weather. A major reason for the popularity of the radiant gas heating systems is the favourable effect it has on the humidity, keeping it at the correct figure.

Ventilation rates

The ventilation rates that are provided in a controlled environment must be considered with great care. In general, many intensive units would benefit from *extra* ventilation. Maximum rates have been raised in recent years to help counteract and perhaps eliminate the overall challenging effects of disease in large intensive units. For layers in cages or other intensive systems the maximum of 6 m³/hour/kg bodyweight (1.5 ft³/min/lb bodyweight) is recommended. Note that the ventilation is based on the bird and its weight rather than the house itself, and the rather old fashioned concept of describing ventilation in terms of 'air changes per hour' is no longer an arrangement that is tenable as it makes no allowance for the birds housed. With heavy broiler breeders benefits have been found from even higher rates and levels – up to 11 m³/hour/kg bodyweight (2.5 ft³/min/lb bodyweight) were the most helpful in the warmest summer weather. The advantages of higher rates for breeders are reflected in better fertility and hatchability, which is probably the result of improved air circulating round the body producing a cooling effect and better health.

However, there is a second very good reason why broiler farmers in particular should re-examine ventilation rates. There have been spectacular improvements in weight and this has meant that unless fewer birds are put into the building or the killing age is reduced there will be too little ventilation. Insufficient ventilation may exert its effect not only through rising temperature and humidity but also by gaseous contamination of oxygen depletion. The main gases that can affect poultry and which are likely to be present in excessive amounts in the atmosphere in poultry houses are ammonia, carbon dioxide and carbon monoxide. Damage to the respiratory tract, which cannot always be detected if the concentration of the irritating gas is relatively low, may become apparent when the subject is exposed to a challenge from airborne infectious micro-organisms. Recently there has also been clear evidence that the serious condition of ascites in largely broiler chicken is due to a shortage of oxygen in the inspired air (see Chapter 11).

An alternative approach to calculating ventilation rates is to base them on the feed consumption of the birds, since this relates to the metabolic rate of the bird. The maximum requirements of this system are 25 m³/second/tonne of feed per day and the minimum is 3 m³/second/tonne of feed per day. Scientifically, this is a sound principle but since in practice it is a rather more complicated way of stating the need, it has not yet found great favour. Calculations based on the two alternatives do not differ very much. Further details on the practical methods of ventilation are given in Chapter 7.

Vaccination and the environment

The points made about health and environment have a special relevance in relation to the use of vaccination against respiratory infections such as

Newcastle disease, infectious bronchitis and infectious laryngotracheitis, especially when given in the highly effective form of a droplet spray. These are live vaccines, which means that they are capable of giving a good, and to some extent an immediate, protection but they are by their very nature, mild forms of infection, so that the side-effects can only be eliminated if the birds are kept in the best environment.

Litter management

The management of the 'deep' or 'built-up' litter in a poultry house is of the greatest importance and seems to be one of the most neglected aspects of poultry husbandry. It is frightening to see broilers, layers and breeders maintained throughout the winter months on accumulations of their own droppings, and in some cases it is possible to have one's boots sucked off in the quagmire – it has happened to me! Birds cannot possibly thrive under such conditions. Parasitic and bacterial infections are highly likely and the poultryman's enthusiasm for the job falls away as he sees the hopelessness of the situation, as no action he can take will materially improve the conditions. Probably the most serious consequences of all are in breeder houses, where wet litter can have a calamitous effect on the feet of the cocks, causing accumulations of infected litter on the feet subsequently leading to a fall in the level of fertility.

Good litter needs care; it is not achieved by accident. A start must be made with adequate material, which can be soft wood shavings or chopped straw, or a mixture of these. Some poultry farmers use shredded paper and 'old' litter from previous crops is occasionally used with advantage, provided it has been completely stacked and heated. A depth of at least 150 mm (6 inches) is required and it should be placed on a dry damp-free base. Studies have shown that litter on an earth base rather than on a damp-proofed concrete floor will contain on average as much as 10 per cent more moisture, so that under these circumstances it may be more difficult, although by no means impossible, to manage. Equally important is the construction of the walls of the house. With an insulated house, the insulation must be maintained to the ground, which is all too rare, as the dwarf wall taking the prefabricated base is usually devoid of it. Also, no damp penetration must take place. In any event, because the edges of the floor are invariably the coldest spots, this is often where the litter starts caking. The consequence of caked litter at the edge of the floor, with birds congregating in this area, is to compound the whole problem, often with disastrous results.

The ease with which the litter is maintained in a friable state is greatly influenced by the environmental conditions in the house, all of which are explained in detail in Chapters 5–7. Above all, uniform temperatures and air movement are essential to good litter conditions, and an even distribution of birds over the floor and modern systems of distribution of the air by diffusion of incoming air are capable of giving the best results.

'Danger' areas in litter management are drinker points, due to splashing or leaking and feeding areas, due to concentration of birds. It is essential to turn the litter quite frequently and often desirable to turn it all from time to time, especially before it is working properly. There is no denying that this is a very laborious task but mechanical implements can help enormously. The important thing to appreciate is that once the litter is 'working' the activity of the birds themselves will keep most of it, if not all, in a good condition. The activity benefits the birds, they obtain some nutrients from the litter and the whole atmosphere and environment in the house can be pleasant. The eventual manurial value of the litter is also increased. 'Working' litter is warm and adds warmth to the house, but wet litter is invariably colder and takes heat from the house in an attempt to dry out.

While it is usual to place about a 150-mm depth of shavings or other material on the floor to start with, it is even better to place a depth of about 70 mm and then add to it as necessary. The smaller the depth of litter that is started, the more likely it is to be totally 'worked' by the birds. If a great depth is put in at once, it is very possible that the bottom part is never moved at all through the cycle, especially with broilers, so that its presence is useless and wasteful. By adding litter later, droppings are diluted, the activity of the birds is enhanced, the condition of the litter is improved and it helps the full use of all areas. Those who have been in the poultry industry some years will recall that when deep litter was first used it was always put down in the warmer months of the year and incubated with some horse manure or other well-established manure to ensure immediate activity.

When litter is heaped, heated and re-used, it is inadvisable to place it in the highly heated brooder area. First, it may present rather too great a challenge of potentially pathogenic organisms. However, more important is the danger of high levels of ammonia from the warmed litter that can result under these circumstances.

High ammonia levels for all ages of poultry are potentially dangerous and are also most unpleasant for the operator. Levels of up to 15–20 parts per million (ppm) are acceptable. If levels go over 40 ppm there may be some reduction in food intake but if levels go over 50 ppm the delicate membranes lining the respiratory tract are affected and respiratory disease is much more likely, possibly even resulting in blindness. By and large it is possible to estimate the levels of ammonia fairly accurately, by using one's sense of smell. If it is definitely 'in the air' then it is really too high, but there are more accurate ways of getting an estimate, either by using a litmus paper colour indicator, or more accurately by using a Draeger gas detector. The latter can detect levels of a large number of gases by pumping samples of the air with hand bellows through indicator tubes that enable an immediate reading to be obtained.

The welfare of poultry

Intensive methods of poultry husbandry have resulted in the expression of a considerable measure of public disquiet as to the humanity of the methods used. The objections come under two principal headings: first, whether we unduly restrict the movement of birds by putting them in cages or giving them little room for movement, and second, whether under some systems we deny them their natural instinctive urges to dust bath, stretch their wings and scratch in litter.

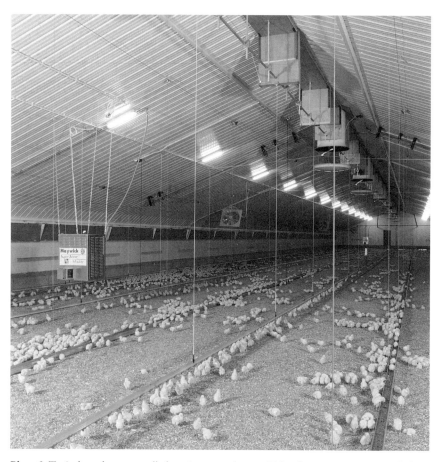

Plate 6 Typical modern controlled-environment house. Ridge fan extraction, suspended gas air heaters, clear span, nipple drinkers, chain trough feeders. (Courtesy Maywick Ltd.)

A great deal of work is being undertaken by poultry behaviourists in many countries to try to establish the validity or otherwise of these fears and it is likely that the questions will be answered in due course. In the meantime, it is important that poultry farmers should be aware of the local laws pertaining to the welfare of poultry. In the first instance it was popular in most countries to rely on 'codes of practice', which is in many respects a very wise way to regulate methods pending the findings of relevant research and investigation. Many of the codes are based on standards that are capable of achieving good productivity and for this reason alone are very worthy of attention. Full consideration of poultry welfare and the use of alternative arrangements to cages and other restrictive systems are given in Chapter 17.

3 Poultry Nutrition

The principles

In order to understand the principles behind the feeding of chickens it is helpful to look at the way in which the birds digest their food (Figure 3.1). The digestive system is simple and relatively short, but extremely efficient. The beak gathers the food material and at its edges are tactile cells by which the birds decide whether it will accept the food or reject it. This is decided on the basis of reflectivity, feel and some taste, although the taste buds are few in number. In certain systems of poultry husbandry it may be the practice to pare or trim the ends of the beak to prevent feather-pulling or cannibalism. Such a procedure may impair the correct selection and apprehension of the food, which emphasises the need to carry out the 'surgery' with the utmost care, if at all. There is no evidence that chickens have any fine or real ability to smell.

The food is swallowed whole, with a little saliva added, passing down the oesophagus to the crop, which is basically a container for bulky foods. Here the fibre is well softened and the food acidified (to a pH of about 4) by lactic acid produced by bacterial action. From the crop the food passes to the proventiculus, which secretes hydrochloric acid and pepsin. This is the organ that most closely corresponds to a mammal's stomach. From here the food goes to the gizzard, a strong muscular organ which contracts powerfully and rhythmically, reducing the contents to a thick, paste-like mass with the aid of any insoluble grit that is present within it. The food next goes through the various regions of the small intestine by the regular 'peristaltic' contractions and it is in this part of the digestive tract that the absorption of the food principally takes place. Digestion also occurs to a lesser degree in the caeca, two blind sacs at the junction of the small and large intestines, the latter being chiefly concerned with the absorption of water. From here, the faeces pass for final evacuation to the cloaca, which is also concerned with the excretion of urine, the acceptance or delivery of semen and the passage of the egg to the outside.

1. Beak
2. Tongue
3. Oesophagus
4. Crop
5. Proventriculus
6. Gizzard
7. Duodenum
8. Small intestine
9. Large intestine
10. Cloaca
11. Caeca
12. Liver
13. Gall-bladder
14. Pancreas
15. Bursa of Fabricius
16. Bronchus
17. Lung

Fig. 3.1 Diagrammatic representation of the digestive and respiratory systems of the domestic fowl.

The condition of the droppings of the fowl is a good guide to its state of health. Wet droppings are either indicative of a nutritional abnormality, for example excessive salt in the ration or rancid oil, or of any generalised 'systemic' infection. Green droppings indicate a liver (bile) disorder, white droppings a kidney infection and red ones show the presence of blood which may be due to either coccidiosis or to an acute bacterial infection.

The basic feeding essentials

Poultry, which are mostly housed without access to soil or herbage and often without any degree of sunlight, must be provided with food which is not merely sufficient for their needs but in which a carefully calculated allowance is made for a safe margin of additional needs. In recent years there have been several cases of the nutritionist being 'caught out' by the very unexpected and high demands of certain elements, often only required in minute quantities. These have arisen more often than not from the success of the geneticist in producing birds with greatly enhanced productivity in every way, so outstripping the normal nutritional requirements.

Protein and energy

The first essentials for the provision of correct, complete and balanced poultry rations are that they should contain the appropriate amount and proportion of energy and protein. The energy fraction is needed for the maintenance of all normal functions and any amounts supplied over and above these basic needs will be used for production, which in the fowl is for eggs or growth. If there is excessive energy in the feed, then undesirable amounts of fat production and deposition will result, which will be harmful to the metabolism and to the marketable product.

The term now used for the assessment of energy is 'metabolic energy' (ME). Briefly, the ME content of a feed is that part which is truly available (or metabolisable) to the animal, after subtraction of the energy in the droppings. Even some of this metabolisable energy is wasted, for heat is produced during digestion and absorption of the feed. The final amount of energy used in maintenance and production is rather less than the ME, known as the 'net energy' (NE). However, it is considered that the ME value is the most realistic value to use, so foods are usually classified and the bird's requirements specified in terms of ME values or needs.

Energy has traditionally been measured in calories, a calorie being the amount of heat necessary to raise the temperature of 1 g of water by 1°C. As the calorie is such a small unit, the usual measure is the kilocalorie (kcal) which is equal to 1000 calories. Now, however, the SI (international), metric system uses the megajoule (MJ), 1 megajoule is equal to 240 kcal. Since at the time of writing both units are still used, the two units are quoted here.

Diets may be classified as high energy (over 2860 kilocalories of ME per kilogram weight of food or 11.9 MJ/ME/kg); medium energy (2640–2860 kcal/ME/kg or 11.0–11.9 MJ/ME/kg) or low energy (2530–2640 kcal/ME/kg or 10.5–11 MJ/ME/kg). High-energy diets may be used for small hybrid laying pullets, referred to previously, so that they may produce the very large number of eggs in relation to their size. Although they may weigh only a little over 1.5 kg (3 lb) they may consume less than 110 g (4 oz) of food daily. Broilers need high-energy diets too as they must reach about 2 kg (4.4 lb) in about 8 weeks at a food conversion of about 1.8, so consuming under 4 kg of food to achieve what are by any standards remarkable weight gains. By contrast, for heavy hybrid and rearing diets the same high-energy diets would be not only wasteful but actually harmful, since the birds would become excessively fat. In particular, the supremely heavy weight broiler breeding stock must be checked from laying too early in their development and should receive an appropriately lower-energy diet to ensure this. In the high-energy diets, the main cereals are maize and wheat, but where a low-energy diet is required the proportion of wheat by-products and barley and oats can be raised in relation to the maize and wheat to reduce the overall ME figure.

Where extremely rapid growth and weight gains are needed, as in broilers, the energy level can be raised by including up to about 5 per cent of added fat in the ration.

Protein is required for the general body development in all growing birds, and layers also need a good proportion in their ration since an egg consists of 13–14 per cent protein. The young chick requires 19–23 per cent of a good quality protein in its diet for the first 6 weeks but thereafter the level can be reduced to 16–18 per cent, 14–16 per cent in the case of broiler breeding stock, where fast growth is undesirable. With heavy type rearers, it is often good practice to feed a supplement of grain with the concentrate ration, but whenever this is done, levels of protein, minerals and vitamins should be adjusted upwards in the remainder of the ration in order to retain a fully balanced mixture of food, the grain being relatively deficient in elements other than carbohydrates. The same precaution is necessary for birds reared on pasture, which are usually fed enough concentrate and grain to provide over half the diet, the remainder being obtainable from the pasture if it is of good quality and especially during the earlier part of the growing season. It is vitally important to understand that birds will eat sufficient feed to satisfy their energy requirements and this is one of the main factors limiting intake. Hence the consumption of a high-energy feed will be lighter than that of a low-energy one and the protein, vitamin and mineral content must be adjusted accordingly in the former type of rations.

The quality of the protein is also another essential element that is rarely given the consideration it requires. The two most important amino acids for chickens, which form the constituent parts of the protein, are lysine and methionine, and the proteins richest in these are those derived from animal origin. For this reason, animal protein is almost always included in chick and broiler diets, although it is not essential for laying birds on medium- or low-energy diets. In some diets, synthetic amino acids are now being used as an economic method of adding these to improve the quality of the protein. The best quality protein of all for poultry is white fishmeal, which may often be included in the rations of young chicks at levels of up to 12 per cent, this amount being reduced as the birds get older. Meat meal products may also be used but often contain forms of protein inferior to those in white fishmeal. The best vegetable protein is soya bean meal, although it is relatively poor in methionine and should be fed to chicks as part of and *not* the sole source of protein. Sunflower meal, on the other hand, is rich in methionine and may be fed sparingly to chicks, although its high fibre content limits the quantities that can be included in the ration.

Vitamins

Housed poultry are entirely dependent on the vitamins present in their compound feed in the correct amount and proportions, and any interruptions in their supply can give rise to most serious consequences, sometimes with striking rapidity. As well as naturally occurring sources of vitamins, an increasing number are provided in synthetic form. The principal vitamins are as follows.

Vitamin A

The principal feature of vitamin A is its function in ensuring adequate growth and as a means of assisting in the bird's resistance to diseases. It may be formed by synthesis in the body of the bird from carotene present in green vegetable matter or yellow maize, or it may be fed direct, either by fortifying the ration with stabilised cod or halibut liver oil, or alternatively by using vitamin A in synthetic form. Chick diets should contain approximately 12 miu (million international units) per tonne of feed, laying diets 6 miu/tonne and diets for breeding stock between 10 and 12 miu.

Vitamin D

Chickens can synthesise this vitamin from sunlight, but even if they are kept under natural extensive or semi-intensive systems, the amount is totally unreliable and usually insufficient for the modern high demands placed on the birds. Like vitamin A, it may be supplied either in fish liver oil or in synthetic form. It should be given to poultry as vitamin D_3 and not D_2, as the latter is poorly utilised by poultry. Unless D_3 is present in sufficient amounts, the bird is unable to utilise the calcium and phosphorous in the diet properly, which are vital for bone formation and for the production of a good quality egg shell. The requirement for vitamin D_3 in the diet is as follows: 3–4 miu/tonne of feed for chicks, and 3 miu for layers and breeders.

Vitamin E

A deficiency of this vitamin causes a disease of the nervous system in chicks known as 'crazy chick disease'. It is also essential to breeding stock for the good hatchability of their eggs. While there ought to be a sufficient supply in the cereals of the diet, this cannot be guaranteed. Also, vitamin E is very readily destroyed by bad storage or overheating, for example if the food is placed under brooders, or by rancid oil or fats in the food. Poultry foods should contain up to 10 mg/kg of added vitamin E, but there is considerable variation between the needs of different classes of birds with the highest amounts required for breeders and young, fast-growing birds. This is one of the most crucial vitamins and in practice it is remarkably easily destroyed between the time it is added to the ration and the time it is put in the feeder, emphasising the need for the expert handling of all compounds and their ingredients at every stage.

Vitamin K

Vitamin K is an essential element in the mechanism of the clotting of the blood and a deficiency can lead to multiple haemorrhage. It is present naturally in all green foods; alternatively, a small quantity of a product which is rich in it, such as Lucerne meal, can be added to the ration, or a synthetic form can be added to compound rations. The needs are small and 2 iu/kg will suffice under normal conditions. It has, however, been widely used by poultrymen as a therapeutic additive, usually in drinking water, to assist in a cure when birds are affected by conditions causing haemorrhaging, such as gangrenous dermatitis or haemorrhagic disease.

The B vitamins

These are well distributed in cereals and deficiencies are normally unlikely, except in the case of riboflavin (vitamin B_2), but the vitamins are frequently added in synthetic form to ensure a constant amount and a safe margin. The main functions of the B vitamins are as follows. All the B vitamins assist the chick in achieving its optimum growth. Vitamin B_1 (also known as aneurin or thiamin) is needed for the metabolism of carbohydrates, while a deficiency of vitamin B_2 (riboflavin) causes a condition known as 'curled toe paralysis' in chicks. Nicotinic acid is also required, especially for proper feathering, and choline is associated with the metabolism of fat. Pantothenic acid deficiency leads to dermatitis. It is also needed for normal growth and for good hatchability and the proper feathering of the bird. Vitamin B_{12} (cobalmin) is required for the development of normal red blood cells and also for good hatchability. It is especially important for young birds and breeders. Folic acid shortage can lead to anaemia and weaknesses of the legs.

Substantial quantities of B vitamins are found in all the following foodstuffs: grains, seeds, fish meal, liver meal, meat meal, soya bean meal, dried grain, dried milk, dried yeast, sunflower meal, unheated offals. However, it should be stressed that vitamin B_{12} is found only in foods of animal origin, or it can be synthesised by bacteria from dung or deep litter. The levels required by chicks (mg per kg of food) for the major B vitamins are as follows: thiamin 1.0, riboflavin 5.0, nicotinic acid 28.0, pantothenic acid 10.0, folic acid 1.5, choline 1300, B_{12} 0.02.

A further important note is necessary relating to the B vitamins. In recent years, there have been occasional serious outbreaks of a condition known as fatty liver kidney syndrome (FLKS) in chicks, especially broilers, which has been found to arise from insufficient biotin, a B vitamin, in the ration, especially where wheat or barley constitute the majority of the cereal fractions and if the protein element does not contain substantial quantities of soya-bean, groundnut or sunflower meal. The total allowance of biotin should be up to 0.15 mg/kg of diet in broilers and 0.18 mg/kg in broiler breeders. Actual supplementation of biotin over and above the levels normally likely to be present in the food would be 0.08 and 0.12, respectively. A major factor in the inducement of the FLKS is when the energy/protein ratio is widened. Peak mortality has been found to occur in diets with an ME of 3000 kcal/kg and crude protein of 18 per cent, a ratio of 166:1, which is too high for the chick (see also Chapters 4 and 11).

Minerals

Calcium and phosphorus

The main function of these two minerals is in the make-up of the bones of the body. They are required not only in sufficient quantity, but also in the correct proportions.

For the young chick the ratio should be calcium to phosphorus 2:1 to 1:1, not outside this range. There is some calcium in all foods, but those of animal origins are generally much richer in it than those derived from vegetable sources. Phosphorus is also present in all foods, but in cereals it may be in a form which is poorly absorbed, so that supplements may be needed. Furthermore, the proper absorption of calcium and phosphorus are possible only if sufficient vitamin D_3 and manganese are present. The young chick needs a minimum of 1 per cent of the diet as calcium and 0.5 per cent as available phosphorus, while the laying hen needs about 3.5 per cent of calcium (approximately 4.0 g daily) since this is the main constituent of the egg shell. Calcium and phosphorus should be added in the correct quantity and ratio, either as steamed bone flour or as dicalcium phosphate, unless the diet contains at least 5 per cent of fish or meat and bone meal. There has been recent evidence that special care must be taken to ensure that sufficient available phosphorus is given, and the level may be increased considerably with advantage. In field trials with broilers, levels up to 0.7 per cent have helped to alleviate the ever-present problems of malformation of the skeleton and the poor calcification of cartilage. Expert advice should be sought before indulging in high levels that constitute almost therapeutic measures.

Manganese

The mineral forms a link in the chain of the calcium metabolism of the bird and is required by breeding birds to ensure good hatchability of their eggs, by layers to give good shell strength and by all growers to promote bone formation. A very characteristic effect of its deficiency is the condition known as perosis, when the Achilles tendon slips off its groove behind the hock joint, pulling sideways and backwards. However, a deficiency of choline can also give rise to perosis and to abnormalities in the metabolism of calcium and phosphorus. Many of the products fed to poultry, such as wheat and limestone, should contain sufficient manganese; if a supplement is required, it is customarily given in the form of manganese sulphate.

Iron, copper and cobalt
These elements are essential for the formation of haemoglobin and the ration may be strengthened with them to ensure an adequate supply.

Iodine
This is normally present in the usual foods, particularly fish meals, but since a deficiency can cause poor hatchability, compounders often prefer to add it as a safeguard.

Common salt
This is essential for protein digestion and is normally added to rations at amounts of up to 0.5 per cent. Any excess of salt, which will result in thirst and wet droppings, must be avoided. There will also be serious deleterious effects on productivity, whether it be growth or egg production, from either an excess or a deficiency of salt.

Water
Poultry have very large demands for water and it is absolutely essential that it is available at all times in all systems of poultry management. Not only will production suffer markedly if birds have insufficient to drink, but in the young chick and in birds of any age in hot weather it may take only a few hours for death to take place if there is total absence of water. There are many ways in which birds can be deprived of water accidentally. Automatic drinkers may run dry unnoticed and this is especially liable to happen with nipple drinkers that have no reservoir where the water can be seen. Also, sometimes the positioning or height of the drinker is such that some birds cannot reach the supply properly.

Table 3.1 Approximate daily water consumption (litres per 100 birds)

Age	Water consumption per 100 birds (litres)
1 day–2 weeks	3–5
2–6 weeks	7–10
6–10 weeks	14
10–20 weeks	18

A relatively new practice is to control the water consumption of growing breeders on restricted diets. This is because birds that are restricted in their feed tend to drink too much water. In programmes of water restriction it is usually provided for periods of 4–5 hours daily, but the procedure advised by the producers of the birds should be followed precisely. Great care must also be taken not to overdo the restriction and very serious consequences can result if the temperature rises above 30°C (85°F) and there is insufficient water available to allow the birds to pant and evaporate off their heat.

Growth enhancers (or digestion enhancers)

At present there are only two growth-promoting antibiotics allowed for incorporation in poultry feed – Flavomycin and Avilamycin. Flavomycin is unique as an antibiotic digestion enhancer in that no veterinary or human antibiotic belongs to the same group, so it is considered safe to use. Avilamycin is also a unique product, being a complex oligosaccharide with the active ingredient Avilamycin. It is safe, effective and has no withdrawal period. Other growth enhancers are probiotics, organic acids, plant extracts and essential oils. A great deal of investigation has been made into their merit and they are worthy of examination by the grower.

Feed enzymes

Feed enzyme complexes are now being incorporated into all types of poultry feeds. The advantages of their use are as follows.

- They have a wide range of enzyme activities in both cereals and vegetable proteins, complementing the bird's own digestive enzymes, being active under conditions found in the gastrointestinal tract.
- They are safe, non-toxic to man and animals and leave no harmful residues.
- They are normally available in granular or liquid forms. The granular form can be included in a vitamin and mineral premix and can then be incorporated in the ration in the usual way for premixes. But if processing is followed by pelleting, particularly where conditioning temperatures exceed about 85°C for 15 minutes or 90°C for up to 2 minutes, then the liquid form should be incorporated at a point in the mixer after the high temperature.
- Their use has given considerable benefits to the efficiency of food utilisation and many help in some respects to replace the use of in-feed antibiotic digestive enhancers.

4 Practical Poultry Feeding

There are several forms in which a balanced ration may be fed to poultry: all dry mash, a mixture of dry mash and grain, wet mash, crumbs or pellets alone or with added grain, plus various combinations of these. All dry mash is especially useful to the farmer who makes up his own rations and because it takes longer to consume it can help to prevent vices such as feather pecking and cannibalism. Wet mash feeding is little used nowadays because of the labour involved (it must be made up freshly each time), but birds find it very palatable and it is eaten more quickly and with less wastage than all dry mash. A mixture of grain balanced with mash is very suitable for birds on deep or built-up straw because the retrieval of the grain scattered on the floor exercises the birds, it helps to allay vices and it tends to create better conditions in the litter. Surprisingly, there appears to be little wastage if the general state of the litter is good.

Pellets and crumbs may be favoured in modern poultry-feeding systems as there is a minimum of wastage, and since each pellet or crumb is a completely balanced ration in itself there is no opportunity for the birds to practise selective feeding. Nevertheless, because of the advantages of dry mash, it is likely to be the foodstuff of choice with birds in cages. Broilers are commonly fed rations 'balanced' with whole grains, producing a bird that is marginally less in flesh but more economically produced (see p. 37).

Restriction of diets for poultry

In general, birds, and indeed all animals, tend to eat rather more than they need, especially if they are placed in an environment where there is little else to do but eat and drink. In a sense, over-eating is a tendency to a vice as much as feather pecking or vent pecking. Apart from the economic undesirability of this, it may also make the birds too fat, or unable to produce as well or as efficiently as they should. If practicable, some form of restriction would probably be desirable after an age of 4–5 weeks, which would be beneficial both for the birds and for food conversion efficiency. Methods of restriction are currently being investigated and there is still conflicting evidence both on their value and the best technique. In rearing, it seems most likely that a restriction of the quantity of the food actually consumed is the best way. Other methods exist that are apparently not so good. For example, the time for which the birds have access to food can be limited, but the birds may learn to consume larger quantities in a shorter period, so effectively defeating the technique! An alternative is to lower the energy value of the food, but this may not be economical because the birds overfeed to compensate, as far as they can, for the lower energy. Yet another procedure reduces the protein and/or the amino acid content of the food; the particular amino acid being lowered is generally lysine. While this method can be successful, it may lead to birds consuming more food merely to correct the imbalance deliberately engineered. Therefore, it appears that restriction of a properly balanced diet by the administration of known quantities is the best technique.

The prospect of food saving in laying birds is even greater, but the risks are also inherently greater if the wrong method is used or the wrong quantities or birds are involved. The effects are potentially good; egg numbers should not be reduced but weight may be marginally less. Food conversion in particular is improved, but there will be some reduction in body weight. The best savings should be with the heavier strains, the least with the lightest, where it may not be a desirable process at all.

There are several practical techniques of dealing with food restriction in the hen. Probably the best is to give measured quantities once a day, and preferably in the afternoon, which reduces the energy intake by some 8 per cent. The reason why it should be given in the afternoon is interesting in that it has been found that the peak requirement for nutrients is late in the day, especially for protein, energy and calcium. Another way of restriction is to limit the feed to two 2-hour periods, morning and afternoon, which is likely to have a similar overall effect. A rather simple technique is to let the birds have an *ad lib* diet up to an age of about 36 weeks and then allow them no more daily than their appetite demands. A very effective form of restriction, which has been used for many years with broilers, is to give them alternating light and dark periods, increasing the proportion of dark periods as they grow. More details are given on this in the section on lighting in Chapter 8 and in the section on breeder management later in this chapter.

The construction of a poultry ration

The complete compounded poultry ration is more complex than almost any other diet on the farm and few poultry farmers mix their own diets because of the considerable problems involved in doing so – also because the highly competitive state of the feed compound industry ensures the lowest possible cost. Nevertheless, whether or not one does mix one's own poultry diet, it is of great importance at least to be aware of the fundamentals involved in feeding, which form the principal 'running costs' of any poultry operation. In the previous sections we have explained the fundamental diets for poultry. Now it may be helpful to look at the ways in which the diet can be put together.

Table 4.1 shows typical nutrient requirements of some common poultry diets, including the vital factors of protein, energy, the most essential amino acids, vitamins and minerals. This is the foundation on which the diet is built. Table 4.2 gives the composition and nutritive value of some of the most common foodstuffs used in poultry feeding, while Table 4.3 gives the range of normal inclusion rates of feeding stuffs in practical poultry diets.

As well as satisfying the importance of the actual and absolute values of the contents, there must be a correct ratio between the energy and protein, which varies depending on the class or age of bird. For example, with laying hens the ratio between the metabolisable energy (kcal/kg) and the crude protein of the diet should be 187:1. From Table 4.1, it will be seen that for a medium hybrid layer, the respective figures are 2800:15, a ratio of 186.7:1, which corresponds well. Growers require a ratio of approximately 176:1, chicks 143:1 at first, increasing to 176:1 at about 8 weeks.

In the construction of the ration, consideration must also be given to the content of indigestible organic material. A bird's gut, as shown in the earlier section on the digestive processes, must have a fibrous content to maintain its natural functioning. In young chicks this proportion is about 13 per cent, rising to 15 per cent in the adult.

In the young bird the figures given should be followed quite closely, but in older birds a higher proportion is acceptable, even up to 40 per cent. In broilers, for example, where there is a simple demand for one thing – quick growth at as low a food conversion as possible – the indigestible organic matter should on no account go much over 13 per cent. However, in growing pullets where some restraint to precocious growth and development can be important to the development of a balanced mature bird, the indigestible element of the ration may rise to nearer 20 per cent.

In deciding on the formulation, all data given so far will be required and in addition it will be necessary to have up-to-date costs of all the likely constituents so that a completely economical ration can be made up to the constraints given. In the end, a diet has to be formulated that is (a) of minimum or at least favourable cost, (b) satisfies all the standards given, (c) does not go outside the minimum or maximum inclusion rates for any of the ingredients, and (d) represents reasonable uniformity of content from batch to batch. Because

Table 4.1 Nutritional standards for principal poultry feeds

	Crude protein (%)	ME (kcal/kg)	ME (MJ/kg)	Lysine (g/kg)	Methionine + cystine (g/kg)	Calcium (%)	Phosphorus (%)	Salt (%)	Zinc (mg/kg)	Sodium (mg/kg)	Manganese (mg/kg)	Vit. A (miu/tonne)	Vit. D_3 (miu/tonne)	Choline (mg/kg)
Starting chicks	20	2800	11.66	11	7.5	1.0	0.5	0.40	60	1500	100	12	3–4	1300
Early growers	15	2700	11.25	8	6.0	1.0	0.4	0.40	60	1500	100	12	3	1300
Late growers	12	2700	11.25	6	4.5	1.0	0.4	0.40	50	1500	100	8	3	1300
Light hybrid layers	16–19	2800	11.66	8	4.6	3.6	0.5	0.40	50	1500	100	6	3	600
Medium hybrid layers	15–18	2800	11.66	8	4.6	3.6	0.5	0.40	50	1500	100	6	3	600
Breeders	16	2800	11.66	8	4.8	3.6	0.5	0.40	50	1500	100	10–12	3	1100
Broiler starters	23	3080	12.88	12.5	9.2	1.2	0.5	0.40	50	1500	100	12	4	1300
Broiler finishers	19	3100	12.92	10	7.3	1.0	0.5	0.40	50	1500	100	12	4	1300
Turkey starters	28	2860	11.96	18	8.0	1.0	0.6	0.45	60	1750	120	16	4	1700
Turkey breeders	16	2800	11.66	8	4.0	3.0	0.5	0.45	50	1750	100	16	4	1350

Table 4.2 Composition and nutritive values of some of the most common foodstuffs used for poultry

Foodstuff	Digestible nutrients (%)				Metabolisable energy (kcal/kg)
	Moisture	Crude protein	Oil (either extract)	Carbohydrate	
Barley	14.3	8.8	1.6	54.4	2728
Maize	15.2	8.4	3.2	65.9	3322
Maize germ meal	8.6	15.4	9.8	18.7	2288
Oats	15.2	7.4	4.0	42.1	2376
Sorghum (milo)	13.9	8.4	2.5	61.9	3102
Wheat	15.5	7.9	0.9	64.4	3036
Wheat middlings	13.3	12.7	4.1	35.4	2332
Groundnut meal (decorticated extracted)	13.4	37.8	1.4	26.2	2728
Soya-bean meal	12.7	29.5	15.8	20.8	2552
Feather meal	11.5	87.6	–	–	3102
Fish meal	10.0	54.0	6.2	1.6	2838
Herring meal	9.3	63.7	10.5	2.3	3080
Meat meal	9.8	65.0	11.9	1.8	3740
Milk: dried, skimmed	6.6	27.5	0.8	42.9	2926
Poultry dressing plant, by-products meal	9.3	71.5	15.2	0.2	3784
Whey: dried	6.3	10.1	0.6	58.3	2860
Grass: dried	12.9	13.0	4.1	10.7	1342
Lucerne: dried	11.3	12.3	1.1	12.2	1100
Yeast, brewers': dried, unextracted	13.3	37.4	1.6	23.2	2618
Rapeseed meal (extracted)	9.6	34.3	1.7	15.8	1760
Molasses	28.7	4.2	–	37.6	1870

Adapted with permission from the *Nutrient Requirements of Farm Livestock, No. 1 'Poultry', Summary of Recommendations.* London: Agricultural Research Council, 1963.

Table 4.3 Normal inclusion rates of feedingstuffs in practical poultry diets, per cent

Feeding stuff	Chicks		Pullets		Layers		Breeders (and hens, ducks, turkeys)		Broilers (and ducklings and poults)	
	Min.	Max.	Min.	Max.	Min.	Max.	Min.	Max.	Min.	Max.
Barley meal	0	25	0	40	0	40	0	40	0	10
Maize meal	10	60	0	25	10	50	10	50	10	40
Maize gluten meal	0	10	0	10	0	10	0	10	0	5
Oat meal	0	10	0	20	0	20	0	20	0	0
Sorghum meal	0	40	0	25	0	50	0	50	0	50
Wheat meal	0	50	0	40	0	50	0	50	0	50
Bean meal	0	10	0	15	0	15	0	15	0	10
Cottonseed meal	0	10	0	10	0	10	0	10	0	10
Groundnut meal	0	10	0	10	0	10	0	10	0	10
Rapeseed meal	0	5	0	10	0	10	0	0	0	5
Soya-bean meal	0	40	0	25	0	40	0	40	0	40
Feather offal and blood meal	0	5	0	5	0	10	0	10	0	10
Fishmeal	0	10	0	0	0	10	2	10	0	10
Herring meal	0	10	0	0	0	10	0	10	0	10
Meat and bone meal	0	10	0	10	0	10	2	10	0	10
Dried grass	0	5	0	10	2.5	5	2.5	5	0	0
Tallow	0	5	0	0	0	3	0	3	0	5
Brewers' yeast	0	5	0	5	0	5	2	5	0	5
Molasses	0	2.5	0	5	0	5	0	5	0	2.5

Adapted from Ministry of Agriculture Bulletin 174.

the possible range of ingredients is so large, an enormous number of calculations are involved in working out all the permutations. The company compounder uses a computer to enable him to do this efficiently and quickly.

There are various ways of setting about a ration formulation. A simple one is as follows. First decide on the energy level that the rations should provide. Then set the protein level to give the correct ratio between energy and protein for fully effective utilisation, as described. Follow this by checking the correct amino acid levels to give neither deficiencies nor wasteful excesses, and finally set the vitamin and mineral levels.

An alternative approach in computer formulation may be required if the economic level of energy in the diet is not known in advance. First, the nutrients are set at levels appropriate to a unit of energy. Then the weight of mix can be allowed to vary between fixed limits known to result in acceptable energy levels in the diet. For example, the unit of energy might be set at 1000 kcal ME and the weight of mix allowed to vary between 300 and 400 kg. Then the energy range allowed in the 1000 kcal mix would be 3333–2500 kcal/kg. The solution would indicate the most economic level of energy to adopt. If it were 2500 kcal (in 400 kg) then the amount of each ingredient in the formula would have to be multiplied by 2.5 to give a mix of 1000 kg.

Commonly used feeding routines are given below.

Broilers

These are always fed *ad lib* from day-old to finishing. A broiler 'starter' ration, usually a 'crumb', contains 22–23 per cent of crude protein and may be fed to an age of 3–4 weeks. Thereafter, a grower 'pellet' is used containing about 20 per cent protein, followed by 'finisher' pellets of 18 per cent protein.

Restriction of intake by broilers can also be made by giving decreasing periods of light, as referred to earlier.

A rather more recent technique, of great interest to broiler growers, is to feed a proportion of *whole wheat*. Feeding up to 30 per cent saves up to 3.5p per bird at 49 days without any loss of efficiency. An investigation by Barbo Tegløf at the Agricultural University of Sweden produced the results shown in Table 4.4.

In the UK at present, whole wheat is introduced at 3 per cent from day 13, rising to a maximum of 30–40 per cent on day 45. Such a technique requires a separate bin for the wheat, together with an accurate feed proportioner.

Replacement stock for egg production

These are normally fed *ad lib* from hatching to 8 weeks on baby chick crumbs

Table 4.4 Addition of whole wheat experiment made by Barbro Tegløf, Agricultural University of Sweden

0–1 week	0% whole wheat	0% whole wheat
1–2 weeks	20% whole wheat	0% whole wheat
3–6 weeks	30% whole wheat	0% whole wheat
Live weight (42 days)	1733 g/bird	1764 g/bird
Feed consumption, total	3247 g/bird	3339 g/bird
Feed compound	2429 g/bird	3339 g/bird
Whole wheat (25%)	818 g/bird	0 g/bird
Feed conversion	1.87 kg/kg	1.89 kg/kg
Carcase yield	69.7%	71.0%

(18–20 per cent protein) and then on early growers ration (14–16 per cent protein) to 12–14 weeks, followed by later growers reduced to 12 per cent to the point of lay (18 weeks). From 2 weeks onwards, mash may be used throughout.

Grain balancer rations are also appropriate. It is likely that restricted diets will become increasingly common practice in the future, as a means of economising on the escalating feed costs without sacrificing efficiency. Farms must follow the detailed programme suggested by the breeding companies for their own birds as these are based on careful investigation.

Commercial egg layers

These are normally fed *ad lib*, with the exception of any addition of grain. Protein percentages vary from about 15 per cent for birds on pasture in summer to 18 per cent for high-energy, intensive rations. While they may be fed with any form of ration, mash is nevertheless favoured for birds housed in cages. Table 4.1 gives the energy requirement of laying birds.

Breeding stock

The parent stock of commercial egg layers are fed in the same way as other intensively kept laying birds. Extra quantities of vitamins and minerals are given to ensure good fertility and hatchability. Ration for high egg-producing strains should contain up to 19 per cent of the best quality protein.

The management of broiler breeders requires the very highest skill in management including feeding and the directions given by the breeding company concerned must be followed. Table 4.5 produced by the Cobb Breeding Company is a good illustration of the care needed. It will be seen how important it is to control the body weight of the breeding stock. The accepted procedure for this is to use separate sex feeding in the production period, thereby ensuring that the males remain in a fit and active condition for longer, with advantages in improved fertility, hatchability and lower feed consumption. It also provides the opportunity for feeding separate rations, optimising the diet of males and females to help maintain fertility, egg numbers and egg quality.

The basic principles of separate sex feeding are to exclude the males from the female feed track to provide a separate male feeding system. The normal method of exclusion is a grill placed on top of the track, which controls access by the horizontal distance between the bars, allowing only the females' narrower heads to gain access to the feed (Figure 4.1(a)). An alternative method is a solid cover for the track which restricts access vertically (Figure 4.1(b)). Male feeders may be a wide pan or tube system suspended about 450 mm from the floor so that it is too high for the females. Such a system makes it possible to control the amount of feed given to the male and also to provide a different ration, for example, with lower protein and calcium levels.

The overall benefits of separate sex feeding include better uniformity of males and females, improved control of the body weight of males and females, an opportunity to feed different rations to each sex, better control of feed amounts to both sexes and increased fertility and hatchability overall. Also, the maturity of males can be regulated, feet and leg problems can be reduced, and males with the most genetic potential remain in production longer.

(a) Grill

1.5 cm   10 cm   4.5 cm   4.5 cm

(b) Solid cover

Fig. 4.1 Methods of excluding male birds from the female feed track.

Feeders

Both hand-operated and automatic feeders are available. The space requirements for birds fed using trough feeders are:

1–4 weeks	25 mm per bird
4–10 weeks	50–75 mm per bird
10–20 weeks	75–100 mm per bird

The requirements for tubular feeds are:

1–4 weeks	one per 35 birds
4–10 weeks	one per 25 birds
10–20 weeks	one per 20 birds

Automatic feeders are of two main types: the trough type with a continuous chain conveyor taking the food through metal troughs from a storage bin that serves one to four outlets, and a pipeline delivery, which operates by conveying the feed in a closed pipeline to tube or trough feeders.

Although the trough space per bird is important, it is just as vital to have a uniform distribution of feeders as it is to have enough space, so that whatever the position of the bird in the house it is not far away from a source of food. This is especially important in the early days of the chick's life and while it is less common nowadays than it used to be, it is still a fact that chicks die because they cannot find water and feed.

The feeders must also be at just the right height so that the food can be readily reached by all birds, but not wasted. For the day-old chick, a description of the need to place the crumbs on the floor so they cannot avoid them will be given later. When they progress to using troughs, these must be gradually raised so that the height is kept about level with the birds' backs.

Drinkers

Poultry drinkers should be automatic, easy to keep clean, free from excessive splashing and not liable to flooding. The amount of drinker space recommended per bird when troughs are used is:

1–12 weeks	12 mm per bird
12 weeks to adult	25 mm per bird

The main types of trough drinkers have ball valves, polystyrene floats or weight controlled valves. But for cages, and for broilers in particular, a more

Table 4.5 Feeding programme and bodyweight guide for typical broiler breeders (Cobb Breeding Company)

Age (days)	Bodyweight g	Bodyweight lb	Bodyweight Actual	Weekly bodyweight increase (%)	Age (weeks)	Feed/day (everyday feeding) g/bird	Feed/day (everyday feeding) lb/100/birds	Feed/day (everyday feeding) Actual	Ration
7	115	0.3		187	0–1	Ad lib to max 35	Ad lib to max 7.7		**Chick Starter** 18% Protein
14	230	0.5		100	1–2		45	9.9	0.9% Lysine
21	400	0.9		74	2–3		55	12.1	0.42% Methionine
28	580	1.3		45	3–4		64	14.1	ME:11.80MJ/kg
35	770	1.7		33	5–6		70	15.4	2820 kcal/kg or 1280 kcal/lb + anti-coccidial
42	950	2.1		23	6–7		78	16.1	**Grower** 15% Protein
49	1100	2.4		16	7–8		78	17.2	0.6% Lysine
56	1280	2.8		16	8–9		78	17.6	0.24% Methionine
63	1430	3.2		12	9–10		78	17.6	ME: 11.23 MJ/kg
70	1545	3.4		8	10–11		78	17.6	2682 kcal/kg or
77	1655	3.6		7	11–12		78	17.6	1220 kcal/lb
84	1770	3.9		7	12–13		78	17.6	
91	1880	4.1		6	13–14		78	17.6	

(continued)

Table 4.5 Feeding programme and bodyweight guide for typical broiler breeders (Cobb Breeding Company) (*continued*)

Age (days)	Bodyweight			Weekly bodyweight increase (%)	Age (weeks)	Feed/day (everyday feeding)			Ration
	g	lb	Actual			g/bird	lb/100/birds	Actual	
98	1995	4.4		6	14–15		78	17.6	**Grower**
105	2095	4.6		5	15–16		78	17.6	No anti-coccidial
112	2195	4.8		5	16–17		78	17.6	At mating change to
119	2295	5.1		5	17–18		78	17.6	pre-breeder
126	2405	5.3		4	18–19		78	17.6	16% Protein
133	2520	5.5		4	19–20		90	19.8	0.75 Lysine
									0.3% Methione
									ME: 11.5 MJ/kg or
									2750 kcal/kg or
									1250 kcal/lb
									1.3% Calcium
140	2640	5.7		4	20–21		100	22.0	**Standard breeder**
147	2800	6.0		6	21–22		110	24.3	(As female)
154	2980	6.4		6	22–23		120	26.5	or
161	3160	6.7		6	23–24		125	27.6	**Male feed**
168	3340	7.1		5	24–25		125	27.6	(if available)
175	3500	7.5		5	25–26		125	27.6	
182	3620	7.8		5	26–27		123	27.6	
189	3720	8.1		4	27–28		125	27.6	
196	3815	8.4		3	28–29		125	27.6	
203	3910	8.7		3	29–30		125	27.6	

usual system is the so-called 'nipple' drinker, which consists of a small rod (or nipple) forming a valve with the metal casing and fixed into a pipe running along the length of the cage or the house. As the bird pushes the rod upwards, a trickle of water flows into its mouth. The advantages of this arrangement are that the cleaning of drinkers is eliminated, the wastage of water is less and hygiene is improved. In rearing birds on litter, there are huge advantages in reducing the dangers of damp litter and there is a much improved food conversion efficiency.

5 The Environmental Requirements of Poultry

Temperature

Brooding temperatures

A traditional method widely used to brood chicks is to arrange a source of warmth in a confined area at about 35°C (95°F) at day-old and then subsequently to reduce this by around 3°C (5°F) a week. Unfortunately, far too much attention tends to be given to the brooder temperatures rather than to certain other important essentials.

In conventional systems the tendency has been to place groups of chicks that are too large under a source of heat with a ring of food and water 'outside' this hottest area. This makes it difficult for the chicks in the centre of the group to reach them. As chick crumbs or mini-pellets are placed for easy access on the floor on paper, cardboard or trays, it may be the water which is more difficult to find. It is absolutely essential that chick water containers of one sort or another are placed so closely and frequently throughout the brooding area that a chick cannot possibly avoid contacting them. Mortality and autopsy records from the poultry unit at Cambridge have shown that in a flock of day-old chicks, on the floor or in cages, the majority of chicks dying in the first few days of life (other than those which are diseased) may do so from dehydration and starvation.

No seasonal effect or evidence of chilling was found, and good access to food and water is the first essential, together with the necessary warmth.

For these reasons, as well as others, brooding systems with larger warmed areas have great merit. They also enable a wider distribution of birds in environmentally suitable areas with more space available, factors that are known to improve growth and reduce the likelihood of disease. To ensure full use of the house as soon as possible, the house temperature is at least as important as the brooder temperature, a range of 25–30°C (75–85°F) being associated with the best results. Above and below this range, weight gains and food conversion efficiencies are reduced. The best performance will probably be obtained if the house temperature is reduced from 30°C (86°F) during the first week to 27°C (81°F) in the second and 24°C (75°F) in the third. The worst results are associated with correct brooder temperatures and low house temperatures – below 20°C (68°F) – when the chicks are reluctant to venture away from the brooder heat to feed and drink. On the other hand, too high a house temperature restricts appetite and retards activity and space heaters should be capable of reaching a maximum of at least 4 kW per 1000 chicks to provide these conditions in a well-constructed house. A maximum availability of up to 6 kW per 1000 is preferable.

If the chicks are to be well distributed within the brooding area, the temperature must be uniform and draughts at floor level avoided. The conventional

Fig. 5.1 Mortalities, food conversion efficiencies and live-weight gains in chicks kept under different conditions from day-old to 3 weeks. Note that the best overall results are from radiant heat at moderate ambient temperatures.

but now rather old-fashioned arrangement of having solid brooder surrounds about 1 m high is generally satisfactory in achieving this and still has a place in poor buildings, but it has been superseded by warming a larger area and reducing air velocities over the whole house. Overhead, largely radiant sources of heat give the most satisfactory results, since their fine thermostat control and adjustable height offer flexible arrangements. They also serve the dual purpose of brooding and space heating. As an alternative, however, blown hot air has its advocates because of its simplicity, low running costs and good space heating qualities. An initial temperature of 31°C (88°F) is recommended in this case which represents something of a compromise between the ideal brooder and house temperature. There should be a reduction of about 0.5°C (1°F) daily until a level of 19–21°C (65–70°F) is reached. All changes should be made steadily and regularly to avoid stress to the birds. Sometimes attempts are made to blow air great distances from end to end of the house, which creates considerable draughts and uneven air temperatures. To compensate for this, it is necessary to lift the temperature several degrees, which can be both costly and unsatisfactory for the productivity and health of the chicks. However, the correct procedure is to avoid this set of circumstances altogether, either by ducting the hot air along the length or width of the house, or so integrating it with the ventilation system that the incoming air is heated as it comes into the house, possibly through a central intake duct under the ridge taking a mixture of hot and fresh air combined. The very dry air conditions produced by hot-air systems are not favourable to the birds' health and well being (see Chapter 7).

Post-brooding temperatures

From the age of 3 weeks onwards, some further reductions in temperatures are justified. In the case of broilers, the house temperature should be in the order of 18–21°C (65–70°F), with a definite tendency to the upper figure if there is any danger of the temperature dropping below 18°C (65°F) owing to external conditions. Under ideal conditions, the best growth takes place between 18–21°C (65–70°F) and certain broiler growers are already achieving this by taking great care that reductions to this range are done very gradually, as mentioned above, so that the change is apparently imperceivable to the birds and at the same time ventilation is maintained without a draught. However, in many cases the heat source does not allow the poultryman to adjust the temperature so finely or gradually, while sometimes the ventilation arrangements are inadequate, with the high air velocities demanding a higher temperature to compensate for the cooling effect. Nevertheless, if the ventilation conditions can be maintained satisfactorily, a reduction of some 6°C

(11°F) between 3 and 9 weeks, gives an eventual temperature of 13–16°C (55–60°F) as desirable for optimum growth.

These temperatures tend to be somewhat lower than those in common practice but their maintenance has important repercussions in reducing heating and ventilation costs and cutting down the effect and incidence of respiratory disease. Obviously such low temperatures cannot be maintained in summer but this is compensated for to some extent by increasing the ventilation and air velocity, if the fans have the capacity to achieve it.

Temperatures for layers

For intensively kept birds, the optimal temperature is quite high – about 21°C (70°F). At temperatures below this there is a depression of about 0.5 of an

Fig. 5.2 Optimum temperatures for chicken of different ages.

egg per hen housed per year per 0.5°C (1°F). Feed intake will be reduced by about 7 g per bird per day for a rise from 15 to 21°C (60–70°F). On the debit side, there is some depression in egg weight, estimated to be about 1 g per egg per 3°C (6°F) rise over 15°C (60°F), but this is far outweighed by the benefits. At the time of writing, it is estimated that if a house is kept at 21°C (70°F) rather than 15°C (60°F), the potential saving in terms of profit margin could be as much as a 20–30 per cent.

It is also as well to emphasise that the hen is reasonably adaptable and tolerant to environmental changes and there is a wide range within which it can produce economically, even if not at an optimal rate. This range is about 5–24°C (40–75°F).

However, this does not mean that the temperature can swing rapidly between these two extremes, since rapid changes of any sort are undesirable. Rather it represents the seasonal extremes one should aim for at the outside in designing the housing in the case of less intensive systems than cages, such as deep litter and barn systems. Provided the changes take place gradually, birds can acclimatise themselves to them. For short-term variation as between day and night, a maximum of 6°C (11°F) is a good aim.

If the temperature rises above 24°C (75°F) for lengthy periods, the total number of eggs laid and their weight and quality will certainly suffer. Appetite will also fall. Below 5°C (40°F) the chief effect will be a sharply rising appetite, although egg weight and quality can benefit slightly. It may be possible to compensate for the falling appetite at high temperatures by increasing the essential nutrients in the ration and so produce as many eggs of almost as high quality on a reduced and hence more economical quality of food. At present however, compounders' rations are geared to the 5–24°C (40–75°F) range.

In order to obtain the required temperature conditions in a temperate climate such as the UK, it is usual to rely upon an excellent standard of thermal insulation and controlled ventilation (see Chapter 6). During cold spells it may be worthwhile to have supplementary heating to ensure a minimum of 5°C (40°F) in deep-litter houses, but it is unlikely to be necessary with commercial layers in multi-bird cages since their body heat will enable a temperature difference of up to about 20°C (30°F), or sometimes more, to be maintained. On the other hand, with deep-litter housing and especially with breeding stock where the density of stock is very low, the combined heat from the stock and the litter can maintain a temperature inside the house often only about 6°C (11°F) above the outside. Experiments have been proceeding for some years to see if there are economic advantages in placing heaters in breeding houses. From records available for study in a number of breeding and commercial egg-laying deep-litter houses, it would seem that the evidence favours the use of heaters in the former but not in the latter. However, as fuel costs show a tendency to rise constantly, the wisest course for a poultry owner to take where there are heat loss problems is to take appropriate measures to improve the thermal insulation and tighten up on ventilation control.

The humidity of the air

There is no reason to have a dogmatically set range for the humidity of the air, although in practical terms the aim in the winter months will be to keep the relative humidity below about 80 per cent of saturation and preferably nearer to a maximum of 75 per cent. If the advice given in the section on thermal insulation and ventilation rates is followed, this should be possible.

In the normal way there need be no problems with chickens if the relative humidity is low, but this is not true if the birds are suffering from respiratory disease (see Chapter 11), and thus the evidence is that a humidity below 50 per cent, especially if it goes as low as 30 per cent, may aggravate infection and help contagion. Infectious particles stay suspended and viable for longer periods in dry, dusty air. It is mainly for this reason that nowadays higher ventilation rates are advised for summer, because while it is not usually practicable to consider humidifying the air to deal with this problem, the dilution of infection and prevention of high dust content of the atmosphere can be dealt with indirectly by increased air change rates.

Water cooling

Problems sometimes occur in temperate climates, and often in hot climates, if buildings become overheated either momentarily or for quite long periods. This may sometimes arise from poor thermal insulation of the building or there may be insufficient fans or they may be operating inefficiently, as so many do. If these obvious faults cannot be corrected, or in cases where after this it is still too warm, there are several ways of using water to cool the building.

A simple device is to spray water over the roof and walls, thereby cooling by evaporation; in some cases a perforated water pipe is placed along the roof ridge to discharge water uniformly along the length of the roof. A more usual way is to pass the incoming air through porous wet pads; the pads may consist of a wooden frame filled with absorbent wood fibres with water falling through from top to bottom. Surplus water has to be collected and recirculated to be economical and the pads must be kept clean if they are to function effectively.

A better way is to have spray nozzles which produce a very fine mist. However, they do need a pump and run-off for surplus water.

A fourth and perhaps the best of all methods consists of a metal disc revolving at high speed which throws off water on to an atomising plate, which sets up a very fine mist taken up by the air stream. Good control is achievable by a solenoid valve activated by a humidistat. Full consideration of poultry keeping in hot climates is given in Chapter 16.

Lighting requirements

In nature, the development of the reproductive (egg-laying) organ is stimulated by increasing amounts of daylight, as in spring, but is depressed when this is reduced, as in autumn. The modern genetically improved layer, under the stimulus of spring-like conditions, will lay before sufficient bodily development has taken place to fully support egg production and it will not be able to lay either the number of eggs or the larger sizes of which it would later be capable. An autumnal pattern, or even a constant day length, will allow the body to develop properly before the birds start laying. Thereafter, to stimulate maximum production, the procedure is to give a weekly increase of light duration of about 20 minutes up to a maximum of 16–18 hours. Artificial lighting is of course essential if this is to be achieved at all seasons, although by rearing chicks in the autumn, the natural advantage of seasonal changes can be utilised.

There are a number of similar techniques used to get the most favourable response but each breeder tends to suggest something different for his own stock, based on sound practical experience. Two programmes are given below for a well-known commercial hybrid. It is noteworthy that the maximum amount of light in 1 day is given as 18 hours. However, many poultrymen prefer to go no further than 16 hours of light in a day, keeping an extra boost if egg production shows signs of tailing-off.

A suggested lighting programme for commercial hybrid layers is:

0–1 week	18 hours light/6 hours darkness.
2–18 weeks	6 hours light/18 hours darkness.
19–22 weeks	Increase light by 45 minutes per week to give a good stimulus at the first period of laying.
23–49 weeks	Increase light by 20 minutes per week.
49 weeks onwards	The lighting is kept steady at 18 hours light per day.

A more interesting lighting technique is the use of ahemeral lighting cycles. These are daily light cycles greater or less than 24 hours. They are not capable of altering egg output but they can improve egg weight and shell strength so that there can be economic advantages to the farmer if prices for larger eggs are suitably favourable. The number of second quality eggs can also be reduced. A 28-hour light cycle using bright and then dimmed lights has real advantages. The dim lights enable egg collections and stock inspections at any time even during the birds' night period; the bright lights have 30 times more intensity than the dim and this stimulates 'day' (bright) and 'night' (dim). A suitable ahemeral lighting programme as devised by the Poultry Department of the North of Scotland College of Agriculture is shown in Figure 5.3.

For broilers, the usual pattern throughout most of the industry is to have 23 hours lighting and at least 1 hour of darkness in each 24-hour period, the latter being necessary to train the birds to darkness. If this is not done and the lights are suddenly withdrawn for some reason, a 'pile-up' is a likely consequence, the birds tending to crowd into corners, on top of each other, so that many may suffocate.

There is, however, an increasing interest in growing broilers on a variety of intermittent lighting patterns, which were once popular, as they appear capable of some improvement in growth rates but more particularly in the food conversion efficiency. They are capable of improving digestion with suitable rest periods, decreasing activity and reducing 'boredom eating'. There will also be a reduction in electricity usage, resulting in at least a marginal saving.

A suitable lighting pattern would be as follows:

0–3 weeks	Continuous lighting (with 1 in 24 hours off).
3–5 weeks	3 hours on and 1 hour off.
5–7 weeks	2 hours on and 2 hours off.
7 weeks onwards	1 hour on and 3 hours off.

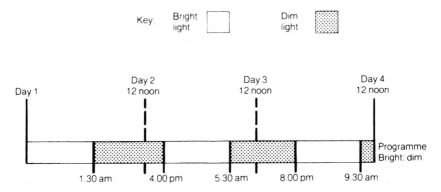

Fig. 5.3 Lighting programme for the 28-hour ahemeral light cycles.

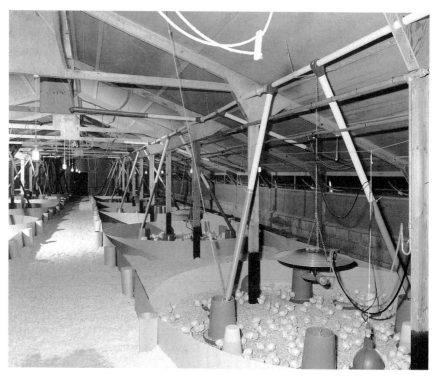

Plate 7 Very young turkey poults under radiant gas brooders with brooder surrounds made of cardboard or hardboard to ensure that birds stay close to the heat, feed and water. Note automatic pan feeders and drinkers. (Courtesy Maywick Ltd.)

If intermittent lighting programmes are used it is vital that the highest amount of feed and drinker space availability must be provided, as the pressure will be much greater on both than with continuous programmes.

Continuous lighting for broilers can be with a light intensity as low as 0.2 lux, which is about as low as the 'off phase' in a controlled environment house in the daytime.

The lighting procedure

For proper artificial control of lighting, exclusion of all natural light must be complete. Fully efficient baffles under fan shafts or air inlet hoods and around the edges of ventilators are essential. Various techniques are shown in the chapter on ventilation (Chapter 7), and it is pertinent to stress that methods used

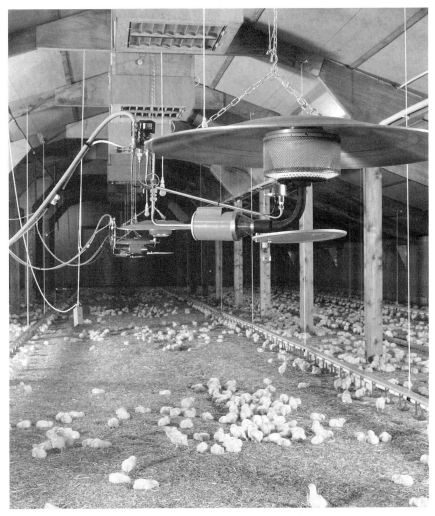

Plate 8 Gas radiant heaters for broiler chicks on straw bedding about 5 days old, with the heaters/brooders raised 5–6 ft high. (Courtesy Maywick Ltd.)

to baffle light entry also serve as draught and wind baffles and vice versa.

The insides of the ventilators should be painted black. The maximum safe level of intensity of stray light entering houses which are supposed to be blacked out is 0.4 lux and it is advisable to check the intensity on a light meter if there are any doubts on this score. For stimulation of layers, the light intensity should be 10–16 lux and there is no advantage from raising the level above this.

If light intensity is uneven in the house, with bright and dark areas, the birds will favour and concentrate in certain areas. This will tend to cause the

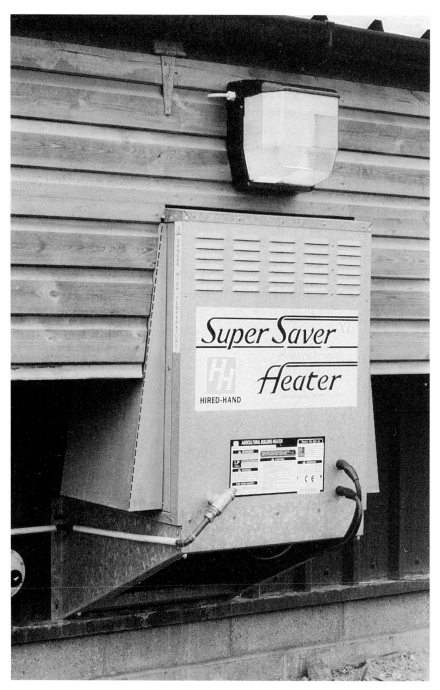

Plate 9 Gas convector heater mounted on the wall of a poultry house to warm the whole house for brooding and space heating.

development of vices and diseases, particularly respiratory diseases. In every poultry house lighting circuit a dimming device is necessary so that light intensity can be lowered easily should there be an outbreak of cannibalism. If birds are to receive sufficient and even light intensity, the disposition of the lights must be uniform. The uniformity is usually obtained by suspending ordinary tungsten bulbs at about 3 m (10 ft) centres along and across the house. A reflector over the bulb will assist in maintaining an even intensity and will help to keep the bulbs free of settled dust.

Suitable systems of lighting which utilise fluorescent lighting tubes with dimming arrangements are now marketed, and while the capital cost of these is somewhat greater than tungsten bulbs, their increased efficiency enables a substantial saving in running costs which can soon recoup the higher initial charge.

6 The Poultry House

Construction and insulation

In most poultry houses, where environmental control is essential, the first need is for a high standard of thermal insulation of the surfaces, which can be absolutely ensured throughout its period of use. First and foremost, a high standard of insulation enables heat conservation to be practised satisfactorily, keeping the ambient temperature just right for the birds and eliminating the use of food as a fuel, or reducing artificial heat inputs. It also permits a levelling out of any wide diurnal and seasonal temperature variations that may occur and, in association with good ventilation, allows a relative humidity below 80 per cent to be maintained. If the relative humidity consistently rises above 80 per cent, condensation may be unavoidable on the inside surfaces, litter will become caked and wet, and serious deterioration of the building may take place. Under such conditions it will be difficult to maintain good health as there will be an increased danger of respiratory disease, and where built-up litter is used, of parasitic, bacterial and especially fungal infections.

The proper way of applying thermal insulation to the building is very important and not infrequently neglected. Many different materials can be used but it is essential that they are kept dry. Apart from the fact that many wet materials deteriorate, they also lose their insulating qualities and raise the humidity of the atmosphere.

While the importance of weatherproofing is generally understood, it is by no means so fully appreciated that it is just as vital to seal the inside from moisture penetration from within the building by ensuring that there is a vapour seal on the warm side of the surface. Suitable vapour seals are polythene-impregnated kraft paper, metal foils and a number of special liquid paints and liquid sealing compounds. Often the matter is simplified, as the inner cladding may also be impermeable to vapour. It is also essential to place a damp-proof course at the base of the walls of poultry houses, as with other buildings.

Materials used for the inside and outside surfaces should be hard wearing and maintenance free. For example, a suitable roof construction satisfying all the essential requirements could be made up from the inside to the outside as follows:

1. Flat fully compressed fibre-cement sheets.
2. A vapour seal of well-lapped polythene sheets.
3. 100–150 mm of glass or mineral wool.
4. An air space so that there is no compression of the wool.
5. An outer cladding of corrugated, compressed fibre-cement or metal.

It is now becoming increasingly popular to use totally prefabricated methods of construction in which sections of roof or wall incorporate all the above features, substituting rigid polyurethane for the glass or mineral wool.

There are huge advantages in such construction, no dangers of vermin within the construction, no settling of the materials and an absolute minimum of maintenance.

Similar methods are often followed for the walls, although in this case the outer cladding is often of timber for the sake of appearance. While timber boards can be used satisfactorily, suitable alternatives are exterior grades of plywood or oil-tempered hardboard. Certain constructions are able to bond the inner cladding, vapour seal and insulation together as, for example, polyurethane faced with aluminium foil or plastic. The final step of boarding the whole roof or wall construction into one place is actually achieved with the use of polyurethane faced both sides with corrugated steel, aluminium or hardboard, usually being used for the exterior surface. There seems little doubt that integrated prefabricated processes like this will become increasingly used in poultry house construction and assist the farmer a great deal by giving a clean, hygienic surface.

Recently, poultry housing has made an appearance with walls clad entirely in plastic sheets inside and out, with vapour-sealed insulation between linings.

Again, the huge advantages in such construction, no dangers of vermin within the construction, no settling of the materials and an absolute minimum of maintenance are apparent. The advantages of using plastic claddings include the absence of maintenance, improved insulation and a generally smarter appearance. However, the initial cost is increased.

The importance of installing insulation properly cannot be stressed too much, and many houses that are potentially excellent are ruined by careless finishing. For example, loose fill insulation must always be fixed so that it cannot slip to leave large areas uninsulated. Also joints between boards must be sealed so that moisture cannot penetrate between them.

The floor is also of crucial importance and yet is frequently badly neglected. Even with a layer of litter, an earth floor can be an obvious place for the build-up of bacteria and parasites. The dangers are greater to young birds. There is no really good alternative to a simple but adequate concrete floor 75–100 mm thick with a damp-proof course between the concrete and the rubble to prevent moisture penetration by capillary attraction from the earth. Careful consideration should be given to the necessary slope of the floor to give good drainage, especially to assist when the building is being cleared out. In deep-litter systems, it is rarely possible to place drains within the house itself because of blockages, but in cage rearing or laying houses, internal drains are of great benefit.

Thermal insulation standards

Apart from the strictly practical aspects of insulation, it is also helpful to know how it is possible to assess the relative insulation value of different materials

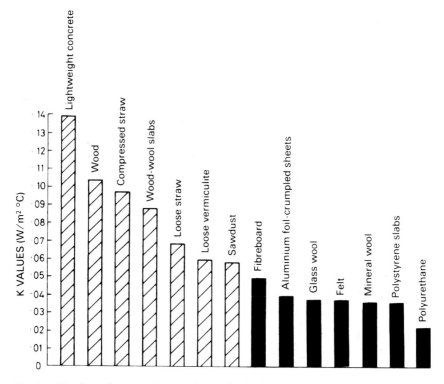

Fig. 6.1 'K' values of a series of materials used for thermal insulation. The sizes of the blocks are proportional to heat losses through them so that materials at the bottom (shown as solid blocks) are the best insulators. Note, however, that a greater thickness of a poorer insulator can readily compensate (see text).

or forms of construction. This will help considerably in choosing the best materials and putting in the right thicknesses.

Every material has a thermal conductivity known as the 'K' value. This figure is the measure of a material's ability to conduct heat and is the amount of heat in watts flowing through a square metre of the material when a temperature difference of 1°C is maintained between opposite surfaces of a metre thickness. It is a useful way to grade materials according to their insulating qualities and goes some way to answering the question as to which are the best insulators. The lower the figure, the better the insulating qualities. A table of K values is given in Figure 6.1 and it can be seen from this that one would need nearly twice the thickness of mineral wool to give the same resulting value as a given thickness of polyurethane. Nevertheless, it may be better and more economical to use the poorer insulator in much greater thickness, depending on the costs of the finished construction.

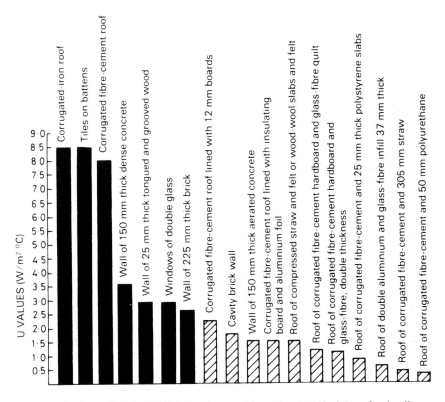

Fig. 6.2 'U' values of bad (solid blocks) and or good (cross-hatched blocks) roof and wall constructions.

K values have limited use because surfaces of poultry houses are generally composite structures. What is wanted is the rate of heat loss (or heat gain during very hot weather) through the whole structure, rather than just the individual materials. This gives much more information than the K value and is known as the 'U' value (Figure 6.2). It is the amount of heat in watts transmitted through one square metre of the construction from the air inside the house to the air outside when there is a 1°C difference in temperature between inside and outside. It is possible to build up the U value of a complete wall or roof structure if one has the K values of the individual materials (plus one or two other figures) but it is unnecessary to do this as U values for complete structures are available from the manufacturers or from technical publications.

As with K values, the lower the U value the better the insulating qualities. A table of representative values is given in Figure 6.2. The striking reduction in heat loss obtained by insulation is clearly seen, the black blocks being poor insulators and the cross-hatched ones are either reasonable or good. These can be used to set a standard. It is wise in most poultry houses to aim for U values in the roof of 0.40 W/m² °C or less, and indeed it is not an extravagance to look for this in the walls as well. The cost of the insulating material itself is modest and exceptionally good value in view of the very great saving it will give rise to in food costs alone. Doubling the standard of insulation in a poultry house need not add more than 5 per cent to the overall cost of the building.

7 Ventilation

Ventilation is concerned with almost all the individual items of the climatic environment, or strictly the microclimate. It must eliminate the by-products of respiration and excretion of the birds, and evaporation from the droppings and its litter. It is also concerned with the control of temperature in the house and humidity, as we have emphasised earlier.

It also has to change the air within the building so that the speed of the air's movement is uniform throughout the house. Considerable variation is required from winter to summer. In winter a speed of 0.15–0.25 m per second (30–50 ft per minute) is correct, whereas in summer, a movement of at least five or six times that figure is called for. This point will be further emphasised in a practical manner later in the chapter.

Most of the modern developments in intensive poultry management have been concentrated on the so-called controlled-environment house, although it is frequently emphasised that such control as the title implies is but rarely achieved! However, a controlled-environment house need not regulate all the elements in the microclimate. What is needed is control over the ambient temperature, air movement, ventilation and light. The standard of construction, thermal insulation and ventilation must be high, but the cost per bird is brought down to an economic level by stocking at a relatively high density. High densities of stock put a very great burden on the ventilation and the design skill required to achieve all these aims must be very high. The ventilation rates are given in Chapter 2 and reference should be made to these for the required figures.

Practical ventilation

There has been very considerable debate as to which system of ventilation should be followed in poultry houses – whether the air should be extracted at the roof and brought in at the sides, or forced in under pressure by fans to find its way out at the sides, or be pulled across the house, from end to end or from roof to floor. It is preferable for emphasis to be given to the fact that it is not so much the basic system that is important, as whether it is a proper design of its type and is well controlled and operated. Ventilation systems should be kept simple and easy for the stockman to *understand* and *control*. Arrangements must always be available for a system that will function should the electricity supply fail, either by designing it so that natural convection can take over temporarily or by the provision of an alternative emergency supply.

It may be helpful first of all to detail the essentials of all ventilation systems. The incoming air must reach the birds at a low velocity in the cold weather; it should also be at the ambient air temperature when it moves over the birds, at which time a uniform air velocity should be maintained. This last point is important to ensure an even distribution of birds on the floor, particularly if they are already stocked at a maximum density.

With the most common ridge extraction systems, an inlet velocity of 60 m per min (200 ft/min) is achieved by allowing 0.5 m^2 (5 ft^2) of inlet area for each 1700 m^3/hour (1000 ft^3/min) extracted. The air inlet velocity is possibly even more important than the air inlet directions, but where the air comes in at the sides of the house the direction of entry should be infinitely controllable, and when the ambient air outside is cooler than that inside, the air should always be directed upwards away from the floor. If the air enters under the direct pressure of the fans, baffle arrangements should be incorporated to deflect it from causing direct draughts onto the birds. If these requirements are carefully attended to, inlet areas as low as 0.18 m^2 per 1700 m^3/hour (2 ft^2 per 1000 ft^3/min) are perfectly satisfactory.

The air should enter or leave the house evenly around the walls or along its length; there must be no dead spots created by large gaps between the ventilators.

The ventilation system should be able to cope in a semi-automatic way with the extremely wide range occurring between maximum and minimum ventilation requirements, a ratio of up to approximately 100 to 10. For example, in a broiler house where a finished bird will require as much as 7 m^3/hour of fresh air on a hot summer day, a day-old chick in winter needs only 0.08 m^3/hour.

In order to obtain the fine control obviously required, it is usual to have a number of fans and speed controls as necessary.

Thus the fans in use may be progressively increased in number and speed from the minimum demands needed for the young chick. There are a number of acceptable arrangements to choose from; important features to look for are that usually all fans are speed controlled and that there is a system for the independent operation of individual, or groups of fans. In order to economise on costs, many poultry farmers try to dispense with these require-

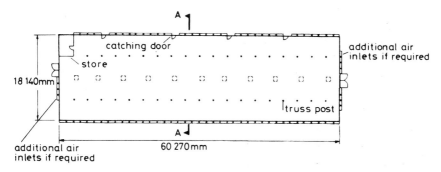

Fig. 7.1 Ridge extraction system with side inlets.

ments but this is a most unwise economy. However, with multi-fan systems, with certain designs it is quite possible to avoid using speed regulators by the use of controls that switch the fans on and off in series. The great advantage of systems like these is that they are economical in cost, reliable, cheap to run and efficient.

The passage of air movement through a poultry house can be studied by using small smoke candles or fumes generated from a chemical such as titanic chloride. The latter type of arrangement gives the best indication of the air currents because it is without heat and fumes copiously on contact with the air. Easily used automatic dispensers of indicator fumes are available commercially at very small cost.

Ventilation systems

The most simple arrangement is to have hopper inlet openings situated along the walls of the building. These are commonly bottom-hinged and open between gussets. The outer hood, with a light and wind baffle, is an essential

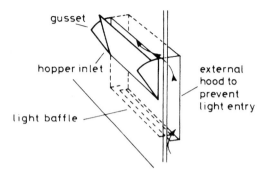

Fig. 7.2 Fresh air inlet incorporating hopper and wind and light traps.

part. On exposed sites the benefits of the baffle in helping to overcome the effects of strong winds is considerable, and is worth incorporating even when the need for such fine light control is not indicated.

In Figures 7.2 and 7.3 two forms of baffle are shown.

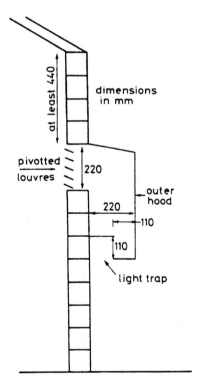

Fig. 7.3 An alternative arrangement of air inlet for controlled-environment housing.

inner insulated
section

louvred intake providing
directional control

air entry
through
slotted
openings

Fig. 7.4 An excellent design of fresh air inlet integrated into the wall structure.

An alternative, more advanced arrangement is shown in Figure 7.4. This shows a louvred intake which is set in the inner part of the wall so that there is no obstruction. The louvres give complete directional control, which can be arranged from a limited number of points. Automatic regulation is also feasible. Instead of a projecting hood, the air enters the space between inner and outer linings at the base of the wall. This means a tidier appearance, less maintenance and better elimination of light penetration and the unfavourable effects of wind.

An important arrangement is the high-speed inlet jet system. The principle of this is to design the inlets so that the incoming air is drawn in at high speed, usually under the ceiling or roof, which must be unobstructed. The air stream sets up a number of secondary circular currents of gentle movement which actually ventilate the birds. The advantages are that the small inlet opening assists in reducing the wind's unfavourable effects on ventilation, thereby ensuring that the air movement and distribution are uniform, stable and predictable. Inlet speeds at the intake are usually maintained at at least 5 m/s, 1000 ft/min. Control devices have been designed to give automatic regulation of the inlet area in harmony with the number of fans operating. This system gives very economical control and is an energy conserver by utilising a minimum number of fans at top speed and by keeping the coolest air under the ceiling surfaces.

With any of these intake arrangements, extracting fans are usually placed on the ridge of the roof. Manufacturers' cowls can be used but as they are rather expensive, the more usual procedure is to place the fan in a square timber trunk. The trunk should be larger in area than the fan, but a diaphragm fitting round the blades is vital. A light trap is needed underneath and the cap over the top also has a lip to assist in keeping light out. Typical dimensions are shown in

Fig. 7.5 Extracting chimney trunk for mounting on ridge, with fans and light trap.

Figure 7.5. A chimney trunk of 750 mm × 750 mm (30 in × 30 in) is used for a 600-mm (24-in) diameter fan. The fan is placed at the base of the trunk in its diaphragm plate; this is in fact the most efficient placing and also the easiest position for maintenance.

In most poultry houses 600-mm fans are used as they are the most economical, although there are special uses for 450-mm diameter fans and for 750- and 350-mm diameter units.

Fig. 7.6 Under-floor ducting for entry of fresh air under battery cages.

Fig. 7.7 Pressurised reverse-flow ventilation. Air entering either through ceiling strip intakes or glass-fibre.

If there is a power failure, the trunks serve as straightforward static extractors and save the house from becoming disastrously hot and under-ventilated. In any sizeable unit, a stand-by generator is best to cope with a power failure, and with most other systems of ventilation it is an essential part of the enterprise.

The conventional system of ventilation described here remains suitable for buildings up to about 16 m (50 ft) span, whether the fans are placed for ridge extraction with the inlets on each side of the house or for cross ventilation with the inlets on one side only and the extracting fans on the opposite side. The system is also suitable for birds in tiered cages when up to three rows are used. However with four or more rows, the outer cages tend to produce a barrier preventing air from reaching the centre and making additional inlets necessary.

One way of providing them is either to place ducts under the floor to open under the central cages (Figure 7.6) or to raise the whole floor off the ground so that the air can enter under the central rows. Alternatively, ceiling inlets by strip gaps or areas of glass-fibre which bring air down between the central rows can be installed (Figure 7.7). Yet a third arrangement has been used very successfully in cage laying houses of up to approximately 30 m (100 ft) in length with the air being blown from end to end. It is pertinent to emphasise that in all cage laying houses, a satisfactory air flow is more likely to result if the passages between the cages are adequate. A 1.3-m (4-ft) passageway is ideal in this respect.

In certain cases, such as wide-span houses and deep-pit houses with stair-step (Californian) or flat-deck cages (see Chapter 9), the air is brought in through the ridge and extracting fans may be placed in the wall. The design of the inlet at the ridge is of great importance to prevent cold down-draughts

Fig. 7.8 Reversed air flow with ridge intake suitable for wide-span and Californian cage systems.

Fig. 7.9 Ridge air-intake.

on the birds. One way of avoiding the draughts is to place inlet chimneys on the roof (see Figures 7.8 and 7.9) with the air passing into them at not more than 243 m/min (800 ft/min) (inlet area about 0.054 m^2 (1.5 ft^2) per 1700 m^3/hour (1000 ft^3/mm) extracted). A less costly arrangement is to use an open ridge with baffle board underneath (Figures 7.10 and 7.11). This may be fixed in position, which is a simple unsophisticated arrangement, or may be controllable both in area and direction so that different degrees of opening and different arrangements for the deflection of the air can be achieved. Downward turned fan boxes, as in Figure 7.10, may be protected from the adverse effect of the wind by the use of a suitable windbreak, as depicted in Figure 7.11.

A more complex technique for air entry is to place louvred openings in each gable end and to run a duct of perforated hardboard along the entire ridge length (Figure 7.12). This serves as the inlet and diffuses the air. Warm air

Fig. 7.10 Ridge inlet system with wall extracting fans.

Fig. 7.11 Enlarged detail of wall hood.

may be injected into the duct if required; for example, in breeding or brood-ing houses. Great care has to be exercised on the detailed choice of the type of perforated hardboard and the correct size and shape of duct, which can only be determined for each specific form of house. In general, a hardboard duct with as large an orifice as possible should be used, and duct dimensions must be such that air does not pass it at much more than 300 m (1000 ft) per minute

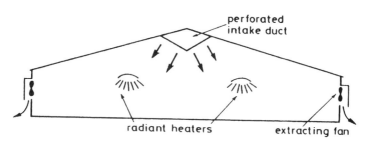

Fig. 7.12 Ventilation by perforated intake duct: louvred gable inlets.

and preferably less. The main practical problems arise from the use of openings so small that they quickly become blocked with dust, or far too large openings that lead to excessive down-draught, especially in the region of the louvres, or the fans if they are placed in this position.

Air diffusion

A further use of perforated hardboard is to place it over the inlets in the walls to diffuse the incoming air, and this is also a useful way of eliminating the worst effects of the wind. It can be placed either across the base of the hood or at the point where the air passes into the house. With this arrangement, as with the use of other diffusing or 'filter' media, great care must be taken to ensure that the holes or fibres do not become clogged with dust or debris, otherwise the amount of air entering the house may be seriously reduced.

In any system of poultry housing where the droppings accumulate under the boards, such as a deep-pit house, it is absolutely essential to have a reversed flow with the air passing in at the ridge or ceiling, then to the birds and finally over the droppings and out. This keeps the air purer, free of gases and the droppings dry more quickly. While it is still common practice to achieve this by placing the extraction fans in the pit area, it is now becoming more popular to pressurise the house and place the fans on the input side to create the pressure.

The glass-fibre ceiling

One way of achieving a good reversed system and pressurised ventilation arrangement is to use the whole ceiling of up to 50 mm (2 in) of glass fibre through which the incoming air is diffused. It has the advantage that the incoming air passes into the house over a very wide area so that the circulation is draught-free and uniform. The degree of pressurisation helps to over-

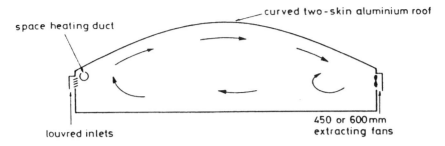

Fig. 7.13 Cross-ventilation used principally in curved roofs of up to 15 m span.

come the wind's adverse effects and the reverse flow makes for a more dust-free atmosphere for the operator. The filtration may have useful health effects by some purification of the incoming air. It is important whenever the roof space is used as the pressure chamber (as in this case) that it is well sealed from leakage of air and it is desirable that it is both lined and insulated. Otherwise there is a danger that, during warm and very sunny weather, the roof space will become so hot that the air will be pre-heated before it even goes into the house. Another especial need is to ensure that there is both an alarm system and an automatic standby generator, as otherwise in such a well-sealed house the birds will very quickly suffocate. A suitable arrangement with good baffle outlet is shown in Figure 7.7.

Figure 7.13 illustrates a very acceptable cross-ventilation arrangement, particularly for curved roof buildings of up to about 15 m (50 ft) span. The placing of the fan on the wall has the advantage that it is easier and more economical to install and service, while an uninterrupted ridge line or roof construction economises on costs. Distribution of air is good and the unfavourable effect of wind is reduced.

A warning must be given. With many of the most sophisticated mechanical ventilation systems, if there is any failure in electrical supply or fan breakdown, there can be little or no air-flow. Thus there is a grave risk of the birds suffocating.

Measures must be considered to install an alarm to warn of failure, and a stand-by generator to take over if there is an interruption of mains supply. In the absence of a generator, a fail-safe system should be provided in which a considerable area of shutters, normally held together by electromagnets, opens automatically when the electric current fails. Great care is needed in making such provisions and expert advice should be sought for the installation of alarms, generators and fail-safe measures.

Plate 10 For wide-span houses the ventilation arrangement shown is favoured with reverse ventilation pulling in the air at the ridge, in this case an open ridge with control flap underneath – and the extracting fans on the wall.

Plate 11 An even better way of achieving the reverse flow. Fans in the gable end of the roof space push the air over a perforated ceiling to give positive pressure flow and uniform movement of air from ceiling to floor.

Plate 12 A similar building to that in Plate 10 but of smaller size with outlet arrangements at the bottom of the side walls. The continuous outlet situated along the walls near the floor is protected by weighted polythene flaps on the outside to remove any chance of back-draughts.

8 Hygiene on the Poultry Farm

It has been emphasised in recent years that there is an overriding demand under intensive systems of poultry keeping for impeccable hygiene. Careful and proper use of a planned hygiene programme is needed to achieve this. Disinfection of a building can take place by natural disinfection and by artificial means.

The disinfection of a building implies the elimination from the house of all micro-organisms that are capable of causing disease, thus implying the conversion from a potentially infective state into one that is free from infection. Disinfectants are the means of achieving this and are usually chemical agents. It must be stressed, however, that a total cleansing is an essential preliminary to disinfection. Organic matter has great power to reduce the effectiveness of disinfectants and without prior cleaning the disinfectant's power can be completely invalidated. On the other hand, if a good detergent sanitiser is used, it has been found that very nearly all pathogens are destroyed, even before the full disinfection programme is applied.

Natural disinfection

Most pathogenic micro-organisms do not survive very long outside the animal body, but unfortunately sufficient may often remain to cause renewed infections. Bacteria and viruses can live for several months if protected with organic matter and the spores of bacteria can live almost indefinitely in the soil or protected in cracks and crevices of the building. Even the coccidial oocysts may survive for years in infested quarters.

The factors contributing towards natural destruction of microbes are nevertheless important, and are in themselves worthwhile aids to the artificial processes. Sunlight, heat, cold, desiccation and agitation all contribute. The ultra-violet rays of sunlight are most potent and their powers of destruction are enormous, but unfortunately they have little penetrating power and cannot pass through glass or translucent roofing sheets, nor through cloud or industrial or agricultural haze. The value of sunlight in animal buildings or on the farm is therefore wholly unreliable. Desiccation from fresh air and wind will also contribute to the destruction of microbes, particularly when the micro-organisms are exposed to these elements by prior cleansing of the building. However, in the protection of poultry houses, and bearing in mind the very short period of only a few days between batches of birds, the effect of natural exposure to the elements is as unreliable a 'killer' as is the sun.

It is also poor economy to leave houses or whole units empty in an attempt to rid them of infective agents; if such a period were to have any meaning it would need to be very long indeed, and even then might be a waste of time. So, the procedure advised (with justification by results) is to carry out such a thorough cleansing and disinfection that it may be considered safe to place birds back into the building within hours of the programme being completed, once the building is dry and any residue of harmful disinfectant has gone.

Traditionally, heat was a favoured method of achieving sterilisation and disinfection, particularly using moist steam under pressure. In farm use, dry heat can be used with a flame gun and moist heat with the 'steam jenny', but both tend to be inexact and uncontrolled methods of applying these agents. For example, clostridial spores may survive heating at 300°C (572°F) for 10 minutes. The very transitory heating from a flame gun would therefore be an uncertain way of attempting to achieve disinfection. Likewise, with moist heat clostridial spores can survive up to 300 minutes at 100°C (212°F). The uncertainty of steaming is thus apparent, and while it is a useful cleansing agent, it cannot be considered a reliable disinfectant when used in buildings where the microbes may be protected in cracks and crevices. On equipment it is more useful, but its powers are greatly increased by incorporating a detergent and disinfectant in the steam or hot water. It must be emphasised again that the presence of organic matter will interfere markedly with disinfection by heat.

Chemical disinfectants

Disinfection on poultry farms is generally carried out by using chemical agents. The lethal action of a disinfectant is due to its ability to react with the protein and in particular the essential enzymes of micro-organisms. Any agent that will therefore coagulate, precipitate or otherwise denature proteins will act as a disinfectant. Amongst these agents are phenols, alcohols, acids, salts of heavy metals and hypochlorites, as well as heat and certain radiations.

Disinfection is not an instantaneous matter, but takes place gradually; however, many more microbes are killed at the beginning of the process than at the end, although there is an initial lag period before activity commences. Also, the activities of most disinfectants increase as the temperature is increased, although there are a few exceptions.

The effects of organic matter

When disinfection is carried out on the farm, almost invariably organic matter will be present. Its presence will interfere with the action of the disinfectant in the following ways. The organic matter may protect the cell by forming a coating on it, thus preventing the ready access of the disinfectant. Also, the disinfectant may react chemically with the organic matter, giving rise to a non-germicidal reaction product. In other cases, the disinfectant may form an insoluble compound with the organic matter to remove it from potential activity, or particulate and colloidal matter in suspension may absorb the antibacterial agent so that it is substantially removed from solution. Finally, fatty material may inactivate the disinfectant.

Approval of disinfectants

In most countries tests lay down rigid procedures for testing and approving disinfectants. For example, in the UK the tests cover a wide range of appropriate organisms in the presence of organic matter. The current Approved Disinfectant Order specifies over 300 disinfectants in the various groups. Those groups that are of special importance to the poultry farmer are Group II, covering those against fowl pest, and Group IV for general farm use, the test organism being *Salmonella choleraesuis*.

Types of disinfectants

There is a wide range of disinfectants used in poultry husbandry and the following information may help the farmer to make an appropriate choice.

Derivatives of phenol, which is not itself used, remain as some of the most popular of all for general farm use. They can act well against bacteria and also against fungi. By the incorporation of organic acids and surfactants expertly blended, their range of activity can also include excellent virucidal activity. Certain products on the market also have other inclusions to give activity against insects, mites, worms and coccidia. These products may be mixed with water or oil and in the latter case the mixture is an ideal treatment for earth floors as the penetration will be good and the residual protection lasts for a few weeks. In practice, many houses have badly damaged floors and porous concrete block wall surfaces that would greatly benefit from such treatment. Such products are specially formulated for terminal disinfection when a complete spectrum of activity is required, since it is safe to assume that possibly every type of pathogenic organism is a potential risk and the specific identities of the pathogens are generally unknown.

For use after outbreaks of coccidiosis, a disinfectant that generates ammonia should be used as this has specific destructive effects on the coccidial oocysts.

Fortunately the poultry industry is well served by a number of manufacturers of excellent disinfectants that provide for all requirements. In addition to the basic materials already mentioned are also aldehydes, amphoterics, chlorines, iodophores, peroxides and alcohols. The user is safe to apply these according to the manufacturers' instructions, confirming that official approval is given, and regarding scrupulously all data on health, safety and disposal. It is advisable to carry out a planned programme of rotating products because all tend to have certain strengths and weaknesses and such a programme will help to prevent a build-up of resistant organisms.

At present, the poultry industries of the world are under the greatest threat from highly damaging viral infection. The enormous sites now established provide a dangerous focus of infections and disinfectants that have a known activity against all the viral families should be used.

Formaldehyde

Some mention must be made of formaldehyde. This is a widely used disinfectant, both in the gaseous and aqueous forms, being virucidal, bactericidal and fungicidal. Formalin, which is an aqueous solution of formaldehyde gas containing 40 g of formaldehyde in 100 ml of the solution, is widely used at 5 per cent strength as a general disinfectant, but it does need to be in contact with the surface for some time to be effective. Its action is greatly affected by temperature and the warmer it is the better, blood heat being most satisfactory. It also acts more efficiently when the surface is wet.

Other than spraying formalin, as mentioned above, solid paraformaldehyde granules are used by placing them on remote-controlled electric hot plates at a rate of 1 kg per 360 m^3 of building space. Formaldehyde pills are also available incorporating formaldehyde plus an insecticide, thus increasing the spectrum of activity. It is rather uncertain how much longer the use of formalin/formaldehyde will be permitted. In some countries its use has been prohibited as a health hazard to humans. Where it is used, always obey the precautions, which are given absolutely by the suppliers.

Control of ectoparasites

It is of great importance to control ectoparasites on the farm as they are a nuisance to both the attendants and the animals. They may be the cause of direct irritation and disease and they may indirectly spread disease; indeed, any infectious agent can be carried by ectoparasitic vectors. These ectoparasites include flies, such as the ordinary housefly, the lesser housefly and the stable fly, as well as mites, including red mite and northern fowl mite, ticks, lice, fleas, bugs, beetles and cockroaches. One of the worst offenders is the lesser mealworm or litter beetle, *Alphitobuis diaperinus*, which is a common carrier of virtually all poultry diseases.

The most effective control of insects is by use of preparations incorporating organo-phosphorus compounds. Such materials are hazardous to humans and must be used with great care.

Practical essentials

The way in which the process of disinfection and cleaning is carried out on the poultry farm very often falls far short of an acceptable standard. Millions of pounds must be wasted annually on the misapplication of good disinfectants so that the disease-causing pathogens quite comfortably survive to re-infect the next batch of poultry. Many of the organisms that cause disease are extremely resistant to destruction, especially if protected by even a minute amount of dirt or debris. Salmonella organisms, for example, have no difficulty in surviving for a year or so and even the relatively more fragile viruses, such as those causing virulent Gumboro disease, can survive for months under ordinary conditions. In addition, the area immediately around the site, which may contain heavy deposits of infected dust and debris, is often ignored in the cleaning and disinfection process. Indeed it is frequently so neglected

Plate 13 A typical group of poultry houses – quite closely packed together and with very easy disease transmission between the buildings, which are only about 5 m apart.

in general care that it can become a quagmire of slime. There are also the active and living 'carriers' of infective organisms, such as the litter beetle. Few sites are without these, and in warm summers their presence becomes greater. Evidence quite clearly shows that they are potential carriers of all pathogenic micro-organisms.

Poultry health and hygiene

To a great extent, the poultry industry has thought that most diseases could be dealt with satisfactorily, or could at least be controlled by the use of medicines or vaccines. In many cases this has been reasonably true. Consider some of the most common conditions, such as infectious bronchitis, Marek's disease, Gumboro disease, Newcastle disease, coccidiosis, epidemic tremor, *E. coli*

Plate 14 Interior of houses in Plate 13. The birds inside will be tightly packed, especially if they are in tiered cages. The photograph shows four tiers of cages, giving a very heavy concentration of stock. The cages shown use belt cleaning daily.

septicaemia – the list goes on, but essentially these are either prevented or treated with vaccine or medicine. Now, however, we are faced with several conditions that cannot be dealt with in such a straightforward way. The new virulent form of the Gumboro virus is not always adequately dealt with by vaccination alone and certainly not by medication. Some of the most virulent types of salmonella such as typhimurium may have to be dealt with by slaughtering the flock. There are also the other zoonotic conditions (diseases communicable to man) where infected poultry, although showing no symptoms themselves, may convey disease to man of quite a serious nature. Three of the most likely are campylobacter, listeria and staphylococci and there are strong public health demands on our poultry farmers to control these conditions. The answer, of course, is to ensure impeccable standards of hygiene, in other words the very highest standards of cleaning and disinfection. Other vectors of disease such as vermin and feral birds, are also known to be dangerous carriers of viral and bacterial infections.

Phases in the procedures

A basic essential is that the cleaning and disinfection programme must be most carefully planned. All birds and all litter should be off the site before the cleaning begins. The amount of infected material that is stirred up and floats around the site when the birds and litter are removed is so enormous that any cleared house is re-infected. I would also emphasise that the litter itself is also vastly infected and it should not only be removed from the site and covered while being transported but should be stacked, spread or otherwise disposed of as far away from poultry sites as possible. In recent outbreaks of virulent Gumboro disease, one could clearly relate site infection from the spread of infected litter. Thus the phasing of procedures will involve clear demarcation of the cleaning and disinfection into four totally separate stages.

1. Birds and litter are moved out.
2. Wash down with a detergent disinfectant.
3. Disinfection.
4. Fumigation.

An overlap between the processes is undesirable, especially for the first two procedures, which are the dirtier ones and therefore more liable to spread infection. There is very much less danger with the last two processes.

From studies conducted recently, the author has been able to establish that the recontamination of a house that has been disinfected takes place speedily and seriously if the cleaning process is continuing on the site. Indeed, it takes place even if there is no cleaning, merely from general environmental pollution. Thus, while it is important to get the various hygiene procedures in proper sequence, it is also important to put the site into production as soon as the houses have been cleared, disinfected and dried. In other words, there is not only no merit in leaving a house empty for a time, but the whole concept of assisting decontamination by having a prolonged fallow period is contraindicated.

Cleaning

There is no hope of the overall hygiene being fully effective if there is any 'muck' left in the house. In the real world of the poultry farm there are not many houses or sites where a fully effective job can be done. This is because there will be basic flaws in the construction, allowing penetration of the structure by pathogens or carriers of pathogens, for example, pervious surfaces, poor protection of joints, wear on floors and inaccessibility of certain parts such as ventilators. There may also be a huge reservoir of potential danger in cavities within the construction. A common area of danger is the cavity between the inner and outer cladding in a prefabricated building. Also, older buildings, which are in other respects often satisfactory, cannot meet with the much greater demands of modern hygiene.

Plate 15 The muck may accumulate in a deep pit under the cages for up to about 1 year.

We have found repeatedly that when the cleaning with a good detergent disinfectant has been done with great care and the muck has been cleared in its entirety, there is little sign of any bacteriological and fungal infection remaining. This enables the two final processes of disinfection – application and fumigation – to give the final near-sterilising effect. The problem, of course, is that in most buildings there are numerous places where it is difficult or even impossible for the cleaning process to do a thorough job. Unfortunately, too, many houses have been built with almost no thought for the hygienic processes. Porous building blocks, poor flooring surfaces, fragile expanded plastic for the roof, dangerously exposed electric wiring and electronic controls all add up to enormous problems, not to mention the almost certain inaccessibility of part of the ventilation system. Some surfaces of the building will not withstand the application of a high-pressure washer so that the only measure one can take is to blow down all the dust and rely on the disinfectant and fumigation to do as good a job as possible. As new buildings replace the old, the modern surfaces and construction should enable a much more effective job to be done.

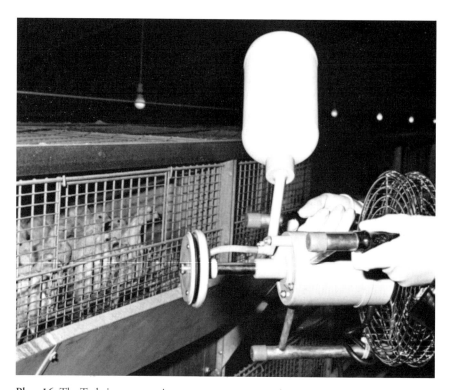

Plate 16 The Turbair spray vaccinator.

In this general cleaning, the surroundings of the site need careful attention. It is clearly best if the immediate area round the houses is concreted so that it can be given the same treatment as the building itself. It is best to look upon it, and also the outside surfaces of the roof and walls, as part of the buildings, requiring the same dedicated treatment.

In those houses with ridge fan or ventilator extraction, a great deal of debris accumulates on the roof and this needs to be cleared off and the site disinfected. If the fans discharge at the side, there are equal, if not greater, deposits on the ground. If they discharge on to concrete it may be cleaned off, but if it is on the soil in a bed of weeds and slurry then it remains a potentially potent source of re-infection unless it is removed or suitably treated. Some years ago there was a vogue for dealing with the problem with a flame-gun but, in careless hands, this turned out to be a rather more effective way to destroy houses than to remove pathogens.

The use of good management of the greensward is preferable, so that the area is attractive rather than being an eyesore.

The disinfection

The house is now ready for the application of the disinfectant. Follow the manufacturer's instructions carefully and make sure that the disinfectant has proven activity against the organisms it is known must be destroyed. These are likely to range from resistant and encapsulated bacteria, such as salmonella or clostridia, to vulnerable viruses such as those which cause Gumboro disease or 'runting and stunting' disease, together with fungi, mycoplasma and others. In addition, special products will be needed for the destruction of coccidial oocysts or for insects such as the litter beetle and vermin. It will not be necessary for these to be used after every crop, but wherever there is a clear indication of infestation.

In several studies done in the hard practical world, the author has found it beneficial to use disinfectants at either double the strength or double the quantity. Many surfaces are very absorbent and have a large surface area to sterilise. In other cases, it is impossible to remove all the organic matter effectively and it is well to remember the temperature effect; most disinfectants are far less active in very cold conditions and this may be counteracted by improving the concentration or the quantity.

A serious point of neglect, left alone to the great detriment of the livestock, is all the equipment, including feed, heating and electrical fittings, feed bins and perhaps above all the entire water system. I have found little difficulty in picking up pathogens at all these points when the usual less than thorough disinfection programmes have been followed.

Fumigation

This is the very important procedure to give a final boost to the disinfection programme. At this stage, the house is set up ready for the next crop and the fumigation can be carried out using a fine mist with a pressure washer or mechanical fogging equipment. The user must be warned that sometimes the most spectacular looking mist fails to get to the parts where it is needed and it is advisable to check very carefully that a proper job is being done by carrying out some bacteriological tests. For instance, in many cases areas protected by posts and beams fail to get much benefit from this process. What is sought is a coating of disinfectant with as long a residual effect as possible over all the surfaces, to see the birds through the first crucial weeks of their existence in the house. There is no real reason why the house – crop after crop – cannot maintain its healthy status if a thorough programme is applied. The first weeks of the chick's life are especially important as it is likely that the maternal immunity is fading during this time and new immunities are being produced by vaccines building up. A freedom from challenge at this time can give the bird an assured future.

Sanitising drinking water

A great deal has been written about disinfection of buildings and sites at the conclusion of each crop and these remain crucial measures. Little consideration has been given to the use of sanitisers administered at a low level as an aid to good hygiene and health while the birds are growing or in production. Yet, again and again in official advice and reports it has been stressed that there is a good way of providing this background of disinfection by sanitising the drinking water.

This requires the use of only very special products. The sanitiser must be effective even in the presence of a fair degree of organic matter; it must be utterly safe to the birds and the operators; there must be no risk of corrosion or damage to the whole water system. It must be known to be effective against certain ever-present organisms in the environment which are capable of being pathogenic to man and birds. Examples are well known, such as campylobacter, salmonella, *E. coli*, including the latest dreaded 0157:H7, and fungi such as aspergillus.

A further important reason for ensuring purity of the system is the use of the drinking water system as a carrier for vaccines and medicines. Important as it is now, it is likely to be even more so in the future as the use of in-feed inclusions of medicines diminishes. The requirement is for an odourless, tasteless and safe sanitiser that effectively removes the 'bio-film' of contamination in the entire drinking system and maintains it absolutely clean by regular usage. Another essential is that there must be no harmful residues created so that vaccines are never harmed when put through the system. Vaccines are fragile and the system of vaccination via the drinking water is inherently wasteful, but the best we can use under the circumstances. The sanitiser should also be capable of use in all areas of processing as well as in special uses, such as hatcheries and transportation.

Chlorine dioxide

A sanitising product which answers this need in all respects is chlorine dioxide. It has been used world-wide for some years in domestic and industrial water systems and especially in those of high danger such as hospitals, and nursing homes for the aged, and all places where especially vulnerable sections of the population are massed, for example in combating legionnaires' disease. It has been most successful as it answers the essential criteria of being safe, it is fully approved by government and water authorities, and is effective without taint or taste, non-corrosive, pleasant to use and economic, being effective at very low concentrations of no more than 5 ppm. This is in real contrast to products such as chlorine and peracetic acid and where far greater concentrations are needed and with a much greater risk factor. In contrast, chlorine dioxide acts primarily through oxidation and is at least five times as effective as chlorine. It has now been used in a number of trials in the form of the proprietary product, Purogene™. Administration is simple, using one of the automatic dosing machines already plumbed into many poultry houses.

The danger of public nuisance from poultry

In recent years there have been increasing numbers of objections from residents near poultry sites who claim that they suffer nuisance from smell, dust, flies and noise. It is claimed that this is not only destructive to the quality of their lives but also causes ill health. Although most of the complaints are rather more emotional than objective, everything should be done to reduce the possibility of these nuisances and the following measures can help towards this end.

It is preferable for a mechanical ventilation system to have positive wall extraction arrangements, discharging the foul air downwards towards the ground. To further reduce the spread of smell and dust, the extracted air can be discharged into a sump containing disinfectant and deodorant with a hessian curtain protecting the fans on the walls. Nuisance from noise can be further reduced by placing insulation panels in the hood; in addition, special purpose-made fan mountings will help further to reduce the noise.

When litter or muck are removed, the trailer should be covered once it is loaded before moving off the site, and the contents taken far away from any danger of causing smell to residents.

Good ventilation and environmental conditions will greatly help in reducing smell. One of the least pleasant occurrences is the smell that arises when there is extremely damp litter in the terminal stages of a broiler crop and when this is being cleared. Good temperatures in the house and ventilation, no overstocking, proper choice and management of drinkers to reduce spillage and a sufficiency of good, well-managed litter will assist greatly. Complaints that arise from nearby residents are magnified if such care is not taken.

Of the greatest help in reducing the risk of smell is to plant a bank of trees between the poultry site and the houses. Psychologically it helps if the site cannot be seen but the trees also assist by trapping the dust and smell and also isolating the site itself from cross-winds.

The flies occasionally associated with a site will be due to lack of attention to the cleanliness in the houses and the surrounds, which thereby afford breeding areas for them. The whole of the site should be kept in the same good order as the houses and herbage cut or land cultivated. Flies may also breed in the dung in deep-pit houses and this may need to be treated with insecticide.

The litter condition can be improved by the addition of zeolites, which are crystalline hydrated aluminosilicates of alkaline earth cations. These have the ability to absorb and control the amount of ammonia and moisture and thereby reduce the nuisance but, in addition, they have beneficial effects on growth and egg production and reduce the amount of damage to the foot-pads and hocks of the birds. There are other additions to litter that make similar claims but they are not widely used, due to their expense. Good management of the environment is the best way to reduce complaints of smell and manure.

Plate 17 Hygiene and disease control are also helped by good roadways and surroundings, epitomised in this illustration of the end of a group of four broiler houses where access is confined to one end of the site, so reducing risks and keeping disturbance to a minimum.

9 Systems of Management

With the imminent and continuing steady decline in the management of birds in cages there is a growing interest in those more traditional systems that maintain the birds in smaller units, often with access to pasture. These systems will be developed and improved to reduce their capital, labour and maintenance costs, which are often high, but here the older, as well as the most recent systems, are described. The traditional systems are not only favoured by a small minority of farmers, but already have a place in the less developed countries. One thing is certain; there will be enormous developments in systems in the next few years.

The rearing of birds

Floor housing

Chicks may be reared on the floor from day-old until they are ready to enter the laying quarters. This is a popular and simple arrangement. There is no stress caused by changes in housing and resistance to parasitic diseases, such as coccidiosis, tends to build up gradually so that the risk of disease from this type of source is reduced. Birds may be reared for any subsequent laying method in this way and it is also a popular practice to take breeding stock from day-old through to the end of the laying period in the same quarters. Some commercial layers are also reared in this way. It can be said to be extravagant on housing as the birds have to 'grow into' the space provided, which must be sufficient for the adult. However, those who use single-stage systems ('day-old to death') are convinced that they gain more than they lose. The absence of early pressure on space does assist in healthy development with a minimum of checks to growth. Both challenge and resistance to disease are favourably influenced as all processes are gradual, and furthermore the labour involved in handling birds and clearing and disinfecting the houses is reduced to a minimum.

With these systems of rearing, a floor area of 0.2 m^2 per bird should be allowed for the lighter breeds and up to 0.24 m^2 for the heaviest birds, the maximum figure being required for broiler breeding stock. The floor area per bird can be reduced by about one-third by using housing of partly deep litter and partly slats or wire. With this arrangement, a useful proportion of the droppings fall into a pit under the slats or wire and the deep litter will remain in a much better condition. Also, by placing the feed and water points largely on the slatted area, the birds are not only encouraged to make more use of this area but water spillage goes safely into the droppings pit.

In those cases where there is a combination of litter and slats, young chicks can be brooded on the slats, which are covered at first with paper bags and litter. After a few days the chicks are given access to the littered area. More often they are brooded on the litter and later, at a few weeks of age, they are trained to use the slats by the provision of a sloping run-up and the addition of food and water troughs to the raised area. Rearing on slats and wire can be used but is very uncommon now as it tends to present husbandry and welfare difficulties, such as feather-pecking, cannibalism and hyper-excitability. Wire with a mesh of 25 mm × 25 mm is satisfactory for all birds from 6 weeks of age, but if used earlier than this a cover of smaller mesh wire is required.

Single-stage rearing is also carried out widely and successfully in special pullet-rearing battery cages, in which the birds are taken right through from day-old to placement in the laying cages. The usual system is to start by putting all the chicks in the top, or perhaps the centre tier, where the temperature can be kept to the required level and where management and observations are most easily carried out. They can then be spread through all tiers within a few weeks of hatching; this change should on no account be delayed or the high density retained in one tier will cause serious problems of uneven or retarded growth. Birds that are reared in cages should be housed subsequently in battery cages and not on deep litter, straw yard or free range since they are likely to have a poor resistance to parasitic infection, having had no challenge at any time and hence no opportunity to build up resistance.

Single-stage intensive systems require careful hygiene, nutrition and management in order to minimise the risk of vices, disease, especially as units may often contain many thousands of birds. They do, however, have the enormous advantages mentioned and they simplify the whole process of management.

Cages are produced that are so designed that chicks can be brooded in them and yet may also serve as laying cages.

As with the floor systems that parallel them, they have advantages in favour of labour economy. In addition, they tend to ensure that the chicks are in small groups, and also parasitic diseases are unlikely and the food and water are very accessible.

Great care must be taken to choose good equipment that has all food and water points easily adjustable and where nipple drinkers are provided; it may be preferred to provide founts when the chicks first go into the cages. The floors may be of 20 mm wire netting or 25 mm × 12.5 mm 16-gauge welded mesh. When the chicks are placed in these cages a temporary flat floor is used, later to be replaced by the sloping floor required for layers.

Multi-stage systems

Several rearing arrangements brood the chicks in a special brooding house and carry them on afterwards, when the period of artificial heating is over, in various other systems of accommodation. A substantial number of these are traditional and often remain in use because the equipment is still available or those who have experience of them are convinced of their virtue. For example, a traditional system is to rear the chicks in a tier-brooder, suitable for the first 3–5 weeks of life. Tier brooders have the advantage that they can be placed in many forms of adapted and non-specialist buildings but as room for expansion is limited they must not be kept in them for too long.

The tier-brooder consists of two or three warmed brooder compartments largely enclosed and placed one on top of another, with runs with wire sides and top and front. The base is of wire and droppings trays are provided underneath. A typical size of tier brooder is 3 m × 1 m taking about 50 chicks to 4 weeks of age.

It is noteworthy that the tier-brooder and the building within which it is housed represent an area of great disease risk because of the quick succession of populations. It is therefore an essential of this system, and indeed of any building where very young stock are kept in quick succession, that the building is depopulated after each batch and then cleared, disinfected and fumigated. The risk is increased further by the high density of birds that the brooder house can contain.

From tier brooders the birds can really go to any other system: wire-floored carry-on cages, deep litter, deep litter and slats, straw yard or free range. However, it is always best to reduce the various forms of flooring used to a minimum, since not only will this result in increased hazards from parasitic diseases, such as coccidiosis, but it will also cause a more prolonged check in growth. If tier brooders are used, a system which has much to commend it is to keep the chicks in tier brooders for a maximum of 6 weeks and then put them straight into laying cages which are specially designed to cope with the feeding and modified flooring required for younger birds.

Outdoor rearing

One procedure, once very common, is to rear the chicks from hatching to about 4 weeks either in tier brooders or on the floor below an ordinary radiant brooder. They are then transferred to a 'hay-box' brooder. This consists of a covered compartment 1 m × 1 m with a run approximately twice as long in front. No artificial heating is required because the covered section is packed round with hay or straw to conserve the chicks' heat and prevent draughts. While the latter part is constructed of solid wooden sides and roof, the run has wire mesh sides and roof. The units are designed to be moved over the ground, which should be good pasture, but they are also sometimes used as fixed units mounted on straws bales.

The system is healthy and can produce hardy, vigorous stock at an economic running cost as no heat is used, but unfortunately it has serious faults in other ways, being labour intensive and with high demands on capital, maintenance, and above all stockmanship. It still has a place though, in the less developed countries where labour is freely available.

After the hay-box stage birds are normally reared in range shelters, or they may be bought to this system from the other systems of management, especially if they have been reared up to then on the floor. Range shelters are a simple, easily made and light form of protection and consist of an ark approximately 3 m × 2 m with a height of 1.7 m at the ridge and 0.85 m at the eaves. A unit of this size will take 60 growers from 8 weeks to about 18 weeks. The roof can be built of metal, plywood, hardboard or felt and wire for extreme economy, the sides being of wire but a large overhang on the roof protects the birds from wind and rain. Alternative housing systems for birds reared on range are the Sussex night ark and the apex hut. The former is a hut of 2 m × 1 m with a slatted floor and solid walls and roof while the apex hut is essentially similar to the other two with triangular cross-section.

A few farmers prefer to rear their birds in smaller groups, confine and protect them and yet still get the benefits of grass. In these cases, the fold unit is the best method. This consists of a hut measuring some 2 m × 1.3 m with a run extending 4 m in length in front. It will hold 25–30 pullets to the point of lay. If fold units are moved frequently, which they should be to prevent a parasitic or other pathogenic build-up of organisms in the soil, the droppings will be spread uniformly over the ground.

Broiler chicken management

The systems used for rearing broilers are probably more standardised than any other arrangement. Almost invariably the birds are reared from day-old to

40–65 days in a controlled-environment house on built-up litter of wood shavings or chopped straw or a mixture of the two types. Because the birds grow so quickly, any upset in the condition of the litter, which must be soft and friable, will be likely to lead to a damaged carcass due to bruising of the breast muscles, which are the most valuable part of the meat.

A typical broiler house consists of a building of 10 000–20 000 capacity, rectangular in shape and from 14–28 m wide. Birds are reared commercially to give a maximum live weight at the end of the growing period of 34 kg/m^2. The lightest weights of birds are marketed at about 1.4 kg live weight, although the more typical weight now sought by the market is a 1.8–2.0 kg bird. Details of the various techniques of brooding, feeding, drinking, litter management, lighting and disease control are given in the relevant sections of this book. It is of some interest to the industry that after the culmination of many years' work in various centres in the USA and Europe, it now seems likely that satisfactory methods are available to rear broilers in cages on suitable flooring of perforated form, although there has so far been comparatively little adaptation of the system. The absence of the commercial adoption of cage rearing appears to be due not so much to technical difficulties as to the enormous capital requirements involved in providing new houses and equipment and also the objections that are likely to arise on welfare grounds. Its advantages would be several, perhaps the greatest being the mechanical handling of birds in their rearing cages to the processing plants, so lessening labour, stress and damages.

Laying systems

Traditional free range

Only a few layers are kept under the traditional free-range system, most now being housed under the modified arrangements described in Chapter 17. With traditional free-range systems, housing is simple and cheap but any real environmental control is impossible. The birds may be housed in movable colony houses of 3.3 m × 1.7 m on skids or wheels holding up to 50 birds. This type of hut has a solid wooden base and is fitted with perches, droppings board and nest boxes. An alternative is the slatted floor house, which is similar but does allow a heavier concentration of stock; a hut of 2.7 m × 2 m holds 60 birds comfortably. It has skids or wheels and is fitted with nests, drinkers and usually a coop for 'broody' hens. Traditional free-range systems can be healthy but it is wrong to believe that they are inherently more healthy than indoor systems. They have serious disadvantages in that the birds and their attendants are at the mercy of the elements and winter production is poor and may even be at a standstill. Some of these disadvantages may be overcome by keeping the birds in a fold unit, as the environmental control is somewhat better. The fold unit consists of a covered-in roost with a slatted floor, measuring about 1.7 m × 1.7 m with a height of 1 m and with a totally wire-enclosed run in front of about 4 m long. The whole unit is sturdily built of timber to withstand daily movements on to fresh ground.

The fold unit has a capacity for 25–35 birds, depending on the type of bird housed. While the birds do benefit from the advantages inherent in keeping stock in small groups and in the movement of them to fresh clean ground each day, the cost is out of proportion to the return. In both these arrangements, production can cease altogether under very severe wintry conditions and it is difficult to see how such costly methods can return to popularity.

Semi-intensive – fixed pen with outside run

The fixed house or 'cabin' with single, or two or more alternative runs, is a system that is only now used to any extent by the small domestic poultry keeper. A typical unit consists of 50 birds kept in a house 3 m × 3 m with two runs each 10 m × 10 m, the birds alternating between them at 6-monthly intervals. The cost of such a system is high both in capital and labour, while the climatic control over the birds is poor. Even when alternating between two runs, a certain build-up of disease may occur. Eggs from this system are often dirty. It ranks as being perhaps the worst of all in theory and in practice but can function in the hands of the domestic poultry keeper where the normal economics of the market place do not operate.

Fully intensive systems

Deep-litter systems

The first really successful and economic method of housing layers intensively was the built-up or deep-litter system. A detailed description of the importance of good litter management in which great care must be taken was given in Chapter 2. After some 50 years of use it remains as a thoroughly satisfactory system, although of high capital cost. Now, because of this, commercial egg layers are but rarely kept on deep litter, but breeders and broilers are. The litter is either wood shavings, about 350 mm deep or increasingly chopped straw; this may be mixed with or replaced by peat moss or sometimes paper shavings but these are rather poor substitutes.

In the earliest designs of deep-litter houses movable perches, drinkers and feeders were used so that, as far as possible, droppings and water splashings were distributed as evenly as possible by moving these around the house. However, under this system, birds require about 0.27–0.36 m² of floor space per bird if the litter is to work properly. It is possibly a cheaper arrangement to have a slatted area over a droppings pit with perches and food and water troughs situated here as well. In this way, the litter receives proportionally less droppings so that the density of stocking can be increased. If the nest boxes are suitably disposed, with feeding and egg collection by hand, the two operations can be combined in a single movement round the house. Automatic feeding is more usual and there are now several systems for satisfactory automatic egg collection, so the 'chores' can be quite well reduced.

With an area of deep litter combined with a droppings pit of roughly equal proportion, 0.18 m² per bird is sufficient for 'heavies' and 0.14 m² is enough for 'lights'. In more recent years it has become quite popular to keep breeding stock on deep litter without a droppings pit but sometimes with whole

Table 9.1 Egg production under different housing systems

	Eggs/bird (dozen)	Food/bird (kg)	Food conversion
Free range	14	54	11.4
Intensive (poor control)	17	50	8.6
Intensive (fully controlled) environment	20	43	6.3

Table 9.2 Stocking densities

	Floor space/bird (m³)
Layers	
Deep litter	0.27
Deep litter and slats in ratio 2:1	0.18
Deep litter and slats in ratio 1:2	0.14
All slats or welded mesh	0.09
Multi-bird batteries and house	0.18–0.27
Totally covered straw-yard	0.27
Rearing	
Tier brooders	0.02 at 3 weeks
Floor rearing	0.09–0.14
Hay-box brooder	0.03–8 weeks
Sussex night ark	0.04 to point of lay
Range shelter *plus pasture*	0.06 to point of lay
Fold units	0.06 to point of lay

house heating provided from an oil or gas-fired hot-air heater or radiant gas heater. This keeps the litter in good condition even in winter. But even without the heater, provided there is very good insulation (see later section) the absence of a droppings pit can be tolerated. By eliminating the droppings pit, there is the advantage that the capital cost is lowered and management, particularly clearing out and disinfecting, is very much easier. It also helps to make ventilation better without the obstruction of the pit and promotes the better distribution of the birds on the floor since there is a general uniformity of the conditions and no reason for areas to be favoured. Because of the cost of fuel, it emphasises even more clearly that the key to the correct temperature needed in a deep-litter house is good insulation rather than artificial heating.

The straw yard or barn system
The 'hen' or 'straw yard' is in essence a much cheaper version of the deep-litter house, using a thick bedding of straw only as the litter and a different approach to environmental control. It was introduced in its original form in the 1950s as a cheaper system suitable for the arable farmer who had abundant straw and a selection of old, otherwise redundant buildings. Because it included a large uncovered yard area, it failed to compete with fully intensive systems since it gave lower yields and often dirty eggs. The disadvantages had to be balanced against the very low capital cost of the system, assuming some cover was already available. One of the worst disease problems that occurred was an infection with intestinal worms, the viability of the worm eggs being favoured by the damp conditions, although if plenty of straw was used and good drainage arranged, the danger could be somewhat reduced. Figures have been produced to show that as good a profit may be obtained per bird from this system as from some of the more fashionable ones but the arrangement requires a high degree of skill in management and has no widespread application at present.

The construction of the uncovered straw yard is simple. The only essential is a shed or yard – uninsulated and open-fronted. In front of this is built an uncovered compound. The whole area is provided with deep straw litter. Each bird is usually given up to 0.18 m^2 of covered space and about twice as much uncovered yard area. Some drinkers and feeders are placed in the uncovered area while the remainder of the food and water troughs are placed in the covered area. It is preferable if the floor of the latter is entirely of wire or slats, on which may be placed sufficient feeders and drinkers, to provide for all the birds in severe weather, but an alternative is to have two-thirds slats and one-third litter. The nest boxes are placed so that the birds have to walk across the slats to enter them; cleaner eggs are produced, so helping to overcome one of the main drawbacks of the hen yard, which is the production of dirty eggs in wet weather.

As the system is intended primarily to make use of existing open-fronted yards, cart sheds and so on, the problem of avoiding draughts and cold winds must be dealt with.

Both the yard and the house benefit from a solid front to a height of 0.6–1.0 m, a cheap way of providing this being to use corrugated sheets placed horizontally. It will depend on the height of the eaves and the overhang of the roof as to whether further protection is necessary. If the eaves are no more than 2 m and the overhang 1 m or more, no further protection may be required.

Usually, however, these ideal requirements are not satisfied, in which case a simple front may be constructed of straw bales and polythene. A reasonably free circulation of air must nevertheless be allowed in the house, otherwise damp litter and condensation problems may result.

At Cambridge we used an unsophisticated form of straw yard for over 20 years which was totally covered but uninsulated and dependent on natural ventilation. This is fully described in Chapter 17.

The slatted floor system

Some years ago, an arrangement was developed for keeping layers on totally slatted or totally wire-floored housing. It is the most concentrated method of housing layers on the floor at a stocking rate of 0.09 m^2 per bird. Labour requirements are low and housing costs can be competitive but apart from the continuing enthusiasm of a very few farmers, who have made it work and still do, in general it has been a failure, with an excessive number of floor eggs, which are lost. Extreme behavioural problems were also created, probably by the boredom inherent in a system such as this allied to the very close proximity of a large number of birds. Nevertheless, in some areas of the world it is still a very popular form of housing, especially in the north-east of the USA, which is an area climatically similar to the UK.

Layout for floor laying houses

The vital feature about the disposal of the equipment in a floor-laying house is to arrange it so that the various tasks associated with management, feeding and egg collection being the major ones, can be carried out easily. In a small building holding up to 500 layers, a service room maybe placed at one end of the house and the nests arranged so that collection is from this room, the nests forming the upper part of the dividing wall between the house and the service room. In larger buildings with automatic feeding, the more usual arrangement is to have a central service passage and nests on each side so that a quick collection is easily made. If the birds are manually fed it is preferable to have the nests against the wall and an overhead monorail and conveyor adjoining the nests. The conveyor can then be used both to collect the eggs and to take the food to the tubular or trough feeders, which are placed on the opposite side towards the centre of the house.

When this design is used in a deep-litter house a central droppings pit is installed and the majority of waterers are placed over this to minimise the harmful effects of splashing. It is preferable if the birds walk across the slats before they enter the nest box, for the same reason as in the straw yard, that it tends to keep the feet cleaner and the eggs are less likely to be soiled. With such an arrangement in a wide-span building, a centre passage would be used with nest boxes on each side and droppings pits immediately adjoining. However, there are those who prefer to site the droppings pit at the side of the house for ease of construction, the usual pattern being to have it on one side with a central deep-litter area and nests adjoining a passage on the other side. This passageway will also take the food trolley if hand feeding is practised. The house will usually be cleared out annually and to assist this the slats, perches and divisions should be easily demountable and the end doors should be sufficiently large to allow tractor entry. Mechanical methods of daily clearing under the droppings pit with a conveyor belt or scraper are used but have not proved popular due to the high capital and often maintenance costs. In fact, the whole trend in all forms of deep-litter housing is *simplicity*, with the omission of any droppings pit and the use of automation in egg collection, leaving the operator free as a skilled overseer of the health and well-being of the birds.

Laying cages

The system of keeping birds in cages from three to six tiers high exceeds all other systems in popularity, world-wide. This is partly due to the breeding of smaller birds which can be kept housed much more densely than hitherto. Also, whereas one bird per cage was the normal practice when the original form of cage was used, it is now the practice to keep between 3 and 25 birds per cage at a greatly reduced cost compared with all other systems, apart from the straw yard. The most popular cage systems house 3–5 birds in a cage. With a multi-bird cage system the *total* floor area per bird can be no more than 0.06 m^2. Cages vary in width as follows: 225–300 mm for a single light hybrid; 300–325 mm for a single heavy hybrid or two light hybrids; 350–375 mm for two heavier hybrids or three light hybrids; and 525 mm for five light hybrids or four heavy hybrids. Cages are usually 450 mm deep and 450 mm high at the front, sloping to 350 mm high at the back. The floor extends at least 150 mm in front to form an egg cradle and the droppings tray or belt, if there is one or the other, has a minimum clearance of 100 mm below the floor of the cage. Each bird should have 100 mm of trough space.

The various cage systems

There are several different types of cages that can be used. The three major groups are as follows. *Stacked cages*, one on top of another, are three to four tiers high and are generally mechanically cleaned by a plastic belt or scraper, or occasionally by using disposable paper belts. A few are still hand-cleared. Occasionally, more than four tiers are used, even up to six or seven, and an intermediate catwalk is required to service the top tiers.

The next group of cages are the *Californian or stair-step*, often called the *deep-pit system* because of the way it is installed. These cages are staggered, as in Figure 9.1 so that the droppings go into a large pit under the cages and can build up right through the laying cycle when they are cleared out by a tractor and a fore-loader. These may also be two or more tiers high, three being usual and four not unpopular. One form of stair-step is the 'semi' form in which the upper cages are set partly over the lower ones, thus economising on space.

Vertical cages   Semi-stepped cages

Fully stepped cages

Flat deck cages over deep pit for droppings

Fig. 9.1 Cage systems.

Fig. 9.2 Semi-stepped cages – great economy in cost.

light proof ridge air inlet
3m APB
100mm x 50mm &
100mm x 38mm purlin

cages

catwalk   droppings pit   fan chamber

section A A

10 340mm

escape door

36 190mm

cages

fan chamber

service area

glass-fibre insulation

3mm flexible wallboard to sides and ends.

D.P.C.   holding down strap

floor bearer, size according to span

foundation detail

A   A

Fig. 9.3 Deep-pit house.

Finally, there is the rarely used *flat-deck system* which is of single-tier cages usually in 2 m wide blocks consisting of four cages with a double line of automatic feeders and belt egg collectors running between the inner and outer cages.

This is the most expensive system but the labour costs can be very low and the mechanical installation is quite simple. Clearing can be either by a scraper system over a shallow pit or the droppings can be in the usual deep pit. With fully automated cage systems, one person can easily handle up to 20 000 birds without compromising their welfare.

Stacked cages remain the most popular. The main inherent difficulties with these units are the automatic clearing and feeding systems, since access to repair any faults while the birds are present can be disturbing and difficult. It is wise not to have too long a 'run' of the belts or conveyors – about 30 m is enough. Manufacturers tend to be too optimistic about the robustness of their equipment under the extremely exacting conditions of the poultry house.

Adequate passageways between rows of tiered or stacked cages are very important for the ease of all procedures. If a unit is a hand-cleaning one then 1 m is advisable. Passageways of 600 mm are general with systems where there is automatic egg collection. While this is adequate in theory, and sufficient in practice, with flat-deck cages it is unwise to have birds so close if it can be avoided. In any system of cage disposition, the passageways serve to some extent as the means of distributing the air to the birds and wider passageways contribute to the maintenance of a uniform, draught-free environment. Conversely, if the passageways are very narrow the closeness of the birds will contribute to the build-up and spread of respiratory and other diseases.

Feeding

The single system of filling the hopper by feed from a barrow is perfectly satisfactory for the small unit but the usual arrangement is to use a system that conveys the food round the troughs automatically. The whole system is automated, into and out of the feed bin and through to the troughs.

Drinkers

There are three arrangements possible for providing water to caged birds; continuous troughs, cups or nipples. With the continuous trough, served by a drip feed or tippler tank at the end, there is the advantage that the birds can see water, have it always in front of them and can physically dip and wash their beaks in the water. The system has the disadvantage that the troughs require cleaning regularly and there is some food wastage. Much more popular now are valve or 'nipple' drinkers, which are valves fitted into plastic piping which the bird can depress to produce a modest flow of water. These are simple, clean and cheap.

Fig. 9.4 Get-away cage.

One nipple is provided for four or five birds in the partition between cages so that birds from both sides have access. Thus all the birds in a cage have access to two nipples and are unlikely to be denied sufficient water.

The cup drinker is a small cup 20–50 mm in diameter filled by a valve which the bird operates automatically through drinking. It is a good compromise between the two systems being clean, hygienic and providing a 'dip' for the beak. There is some evidence that birds do rather better with water in front of them but it is not consistent and nipples cannot be condemned on the grounds of the rather flimsy evidence available.

The 'get-away' cage

Mention should be made of the so called 'get-away' cages, as these have been designed for important reasons. The cage (Figure 9.4) provides three areas – a horizontal wire floor, a nest box and areas for perching. They also have two levels of feeders and drinkers. These are to provide an environment which is rather more akin to the 'natural' state insofar as there are perches for resting (the 'get-away' part), a separate area for laying and extra facilities for feeding and drinking. In this allegedly less stressful environment it is believed there may be less likelihood of a welfare problem and better production, so compensating for the extra cost. A number of commercial developments have been produced and are referred to later, to try and incorporate the parts listed above.

Record keeping

It is always essential to record carefully the results of performance in all systems of poultry production, from which the margin of profit (or loss) can be evaluated. For example, with a laying flock one would take the following records at least:

- The total number of birds housed.
- The cost of the birds or rearing costs if done by the owner.
- Eggs collected daily.
- Food consumed daily.
- Egg sales.
- Grading details.
- Mortality and culls daily.
- Birds sold at end of lay and their value.
- Labour costs.

Most useful calculations for a farmer to make frequently, usually weekly, from the figures collected are as follows.

$$\% \text{ Egg production per week} = \frac{\text{Total eggs per week} \times 100}{\text{Average no. of birds per week} \times 7}$$

and

% Egg production, based on no. of birds housed (hen-housed) =

$$\frac{\text{Total eggs to date} \times 100}{\text{No. of birds housed} \times \text{no. of days since housing}}$$

The latter gives the percentage of production based on the birds housed (hen house average) and is a frequently used figure. A graph of production day by day is invaluable to give a quick check on productivity and is a clear way to detect trends early on. The profit and loss of the farm from time to time can be worked out quite readily from these basic figures.

For broilers a popular yardstick of efficiency is the European Production Efficiency Factor (EPEF), which is as follows:

$$\text{EPEF} = \frac{\text{Av. liveweight} \times \dfrac{\text{Total liveweight sold}}{\text{No. of chicks started}}}{\text{Av. liveweight} \times \dfrac{\text{Total feed used}}{\text{No. of broilers sold}}} \times 10\,000$$

Plate 18 Interior of deep-litter poultry houses containing heavy 'boiler breeders', normally housed at about three birds per square metre. The automatic chain feeder is in the foreground while the self-filling drinkers can be seen at several positions. The individual laying boxes are visible on the partition between the pens. The management of broiler breeders is one of the most demanding undertakings for the poultryman. A good feeding routine, excellent management of the litter, fine control of the environment and constant and careful care and handling of the birds are necessary to achieve satisfactory results. Good management can give up to 140 fertile eggs per bird but under poorer control the number may be barely 100.

Plate 19 Exterior of the deep-litter breeding house shown in Plate 18. The building has reversed air flow, with ridge air intake and side-wall extraction. The bulk food bins are a prominent feature but the overall appearance is attractive, with the light coloured fibre-cement roof contrasting with the creosoted timber exterior. The wall fan cowls are fitted with special devices to reduce back-draught. With sites such as this, great importance is attached to the general standards of cleanliness and hygiene around the buildings since they will contribute to the overall success of the operation.

All measurements are in kilograms (kg). If this seems rather complex, the most important needs with broilers which can easily be calculated are:

1. *Liveability* – the percentage of chicks alive at the end of the crop.
2. *Feed conversion efficiency (or ratio) FCR* – divide the total weight of the feed used by the total liveweight started.
3. *Feed cost per kg liveweight* – multiply FCR by cost of feed per kg.
4. *Average weight per bird* – divide the weight of birds sold by the number of birds sold.
5. *Gross margin per unit of floor space* – subtract the feed cost from the gross income and then divide the result by the floor area (m^2 or ft^2).

To aid the poultry farmer in keeping records, excellent assistance is usually available from national compounders, breeders, hatchery organisations or the government advisory services. The poultryman is exhorted to make good use of these invaluable facilities as they remove the tedium and make record keeping a useful and fascinating job.

10 Breeding and Hatching

In other sections of this book I have emphasised many of the essentials for the production of hatching eggs. The sections include those on nutrition, housing and disease control. It must be stressed that the effective demand on nutritional elements by breeders is especially great. In recent years the production of breeding stock has been markedly improved so that with the feeding of restricted rations it becomes more important than ever that the essential vitamins, minerals and amino acids are supplied in adequate amounts. This will have a profound effect on the fertility and hatchability. Special attention should be given to the nutrition during the depths of winter and early spring when the quality of the eggs and the chicks can often deteriorate. As this tends to be a constant seasonal problem, it is difficult to understand why this is so often tolerated. Special attention should be paid to vitamins A, D_3, B_{12} and the B vitamins in general, and to manganese, zinc and choline.

It is also important to reiterate that healthy stock is particularly important for the production of sound hatching eggs. All diseases have an adverse effect in the ultimate viability of the bird, the eggs produced by it and the chick that may emerge. Some diseases in particular, such as infectious bronchitis and EDS '76, have an almost catastrophic effect, always for some time and often for the remainder of the bird's life (see Chapter 11).

The fertility of poultry is partly dependent on the genetics and selection of the birds as inherent qualities, but is also dependent on good management. A very important feature is the mating ratio – usually the optimum ratio is six or seven males to 100 females for pullet replacements and between seven and nine males per 100 females for broiler breeders. It should be borne in mind that once a group of males are made up, it is preferable not to interfere with them.

Hatchability as well as fertility is affected by genetic factors, but once again it is management that transcends genetics in its effects.

It is vital that hygienic standards in the breeder house are impeccable to avoid infections entering the incubator either within or on the shell of the egg. Nests must be clean and the litter dry; only clean wood shavings or other sterile litter should be used and certainly *never* damp hay or straw. It must be changed regularly and eggs laid on the litter should not go into the incubator if at all possible. The greatest danger is that the hatching eggs will be contaminated with *Aspergillus fumigatus* (see Chapter 11) which may be very difficult to eliminate if it gets into the hatchery.

For the best results, hatching eggs should be collected at least three times a day, and in this way they keep cleaner and can be cooled more quickly. Selection of eggs subsequently is important, removing all sub-standard eggs with misshapen, cracked or thin shells. Eggs that are either too big or too small are undesirable and usually those between 48 and 64 g (1.75–2.25 oz) are favoured. As soon as possible after collection, the eggs should be fumigated with formaldehyde in a special cabinet, although they may be dry cleaned, washed or dipped in specially sanitised solutions at a temperature very slightly warmer than the eggs. Great care must be taken to ensure that the sanitising material is safe and is frequently changed. It is not uncommon for dirty solutions to do more harm than good by spreading infection.

The conditions under which the eggs are stored before incubation need good control. The optimal range is 13–16°C (55–60°F) with a high relative humidity of 75–80 per cent. In order to maintain such conditions, all farm egg stores should be well insulated and preferably equipped with an appropriate air conditioner if the eggs are to be stored for long. Pre-incubation storage should not go on for more than 7 days, but a limit of 4 days is preferable since up to this limit there is almost no loss in hatchability if storage conditions are good.

The actual handling of the egg needs great care at every stage, and this does not apply only to the hygienic measures. The living embryo that it contains is marvellously protected but nevertheless can be damaged by rough handling. Gentle transfer of the eggs from one place to another is required and will subsequently improve the hatchability. The use of plastic setting trays has much to commend it as the trays can be used for on-farm traying so that handling subsequent to this is eliminated and fumigation is more effectively achieved. Plastic trays can be properly cleaned and sterilised at the hatchery and then re-used, where the old-fashioned fibre trays could not.

In the course of incubation eggs are 'candled' – a bright light source is placed under the eggs and on viewing from above those eggs that are fertile appear relatively opaque due to the opacity of the developing embryo, while the non-fertile ones are clear. The 'clears' should be removed without delay, as they can be a source of disease if they remain in the incubator and break.

Incubation

There are two principal types of incubator – the smaller cabinet incubator or the large walk-in mammoth incubator. These are usually divided into two processes, the 'setters', which receive the eggs for the first 18 days, subsequently entering the 'hatcher' for the final 3 days. A few eggs are still hatched in small flat incubators, where the eggs lie flat on their sides, which are usually combined setters and hatchers. These are suitable for hatching small numbers of eggs. Conditions required within the larger incubators are as follows:

	Temperature	*Relative humidity*
1–18 days	37.5–37.8°C (99.5–100°F)	60%
18–21 days	36.9–37.5°C (98.5–99.5°F)	60%

The conditions required in the small flat incubator without mechanical aids to the ventilation are rather different – a temperature of 38°C (103°F) is needed to ensure proper conditions at the centre of the egg.

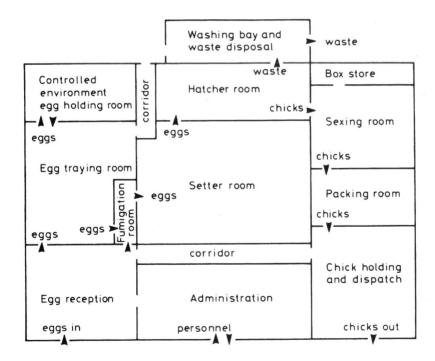

Fig. 10.1 Specimen hatchery layout (not to scale – diagrammatic only).

Any wide variation from the optimal figures is likely to lead to serious consequences. For example, if the humidity is too low, excessive moisture is lost from the egg and many chicks will fail to hatch. If the humidity is too high, the chicks may hatch early and are excessively wet.

In the larger incubators, the eggs are placed in trays with the broad end higher than the narrow end. The eggs must be turned frequently to ensure that the embryo does not settle and adhere to other structures. Turning is usually done automatically hourly through 45° to the vertical. No turning is necessary in the hatching compartment.

Control of the ventilation by mechanical means is always carried out in large incubators so that the critical needs of the eggs for supplying oxygen and removing carbon dioxide are achieved. Carbon dioxide must not go above 0.4 per cent and oxygen must be at least 17.5 per cent. Incubator manufacturers do design all their machines to achieve the required conditions in various ways and their directions should be followed for the best results.

Most incubators are powered entirely by electricity and if there is a power failure high levels of carbon dioxide could quickly kill the embryos. Because of this, a standby generator is an essential for the immediate takeover of power when the mains fail.

The precise design of the incubators – setters and hatchers – varies according to its manufacturer and the whole process of design and management of hatcheries is becoming increasingly sophisticated and complex, and is clearly outside the scope of this book. However, the modern hatchery represents the greatest area of disease risk in a modern poultry enterprise, being a bottleneck through which every chick passes. By its usual large size it is at even greater risk, and we should carefully consider some of the essentials which have a bearing on these facets and which have not already been touched upon.

The incubators must be so ventilated that each unit receives fresh air from the outside and discharges its stale vitiated air to the outside, thus ensuring a minimum of air pollution in the hatcher itself. All surfaces of the building and the incubators must be of the best materials to ensure that they can be sterilised readily and efficiently. In many modern installations, it is appropriate to actually filter the air into the incubator machinery. Within the hatcher, there must be a 'flow of air' such that it can never pass back from 'dirty' areas, such as the hatchers, to clean areas and the setters and egg-holding rooms. In the same way, the movement of people and equipment has to be carefully designed and managed to give the same clean flow principle. Figure 10.1 shows the complexity of the modern hatchery and the various essential parts. Eggs will be received from the farms into the egg reception area, which should be big enough to take about a a day's supply; if the eggs are to be held longer, they must go into a special egg-holding room after fumigation. Fumigation will take place again before the eggs go into the setter. The fumigation chamber should be sealable when fumigation is taking place and have powered ventilation to disperse the gas after fumigation.

It is especially important that where there is a separate hatching area – usually where mammoth outfits are concerned – this is well sealed from the rest of the hatchery. The discharged air which will contain a good deal of potentially polluted material should be collected by traps and/or filters so that there is a minimum chance of recirculation of the extracted air back to the input side.

In the day-to-day management of the hatchery it is very useful to aerosol the atmosphere frequently with disinfectants. Care must also be taken with the staff, who should practise impeccable personal hygiene and should, from time to time, be checked for salmonella infections.

Plate 20 A group of three thermostats giving variable speed operation of fans. There are a number of devices that achieve such control but in essence the thermostat (or thermistor) devices in the house are wired to control boxes of some complexity.

Plate 21 A typical control box which incorporates the 'brains' to regulate heating, lighting and ventilation.

11 The Health of Poultry

This section of the book describes the diseases of poultry, their signs, prevention and treatment. It is in no way intended to be a catalogue or dictionary of diseases, to be available only for reference on those occasions when it appears to be needed, usually after a disease has 'struck' and it is already far too late to control it effectively. Rather, the purpose of this part of the book is to explain the circumstances and conditions under which specified diseases are liable to occur and how, by good management built on the foundation of basically sound units and buildings, not only will disease be far less likely to occur but, in addition, productivity can be enhanced at all ages and stages.

The most useful way for the poultry farmer or attendant to consider the incidence of disease is on a life-cycle sequence and this will be done by starting with the chick and tracing the likely disease problems through life.

The chick

In earlier sections of the book, the management of the day-old chick has been stressed in some detail. There is no escaping the fact that the day-old chick is peculiarly vulnerable to stress, and conditions must be accurately maintained to avoid either chilling or overheating. Unfortunately, as birds are kept in larger and larger numbers in one house, unless very sophisticated environmental control systems are used it is almost impossible to provide a uniform environment. While the conditions required by the chick are well known, the ability of the housing to provide them properly is often lacking. Thus there may be almost immediate losses from chilling in certain areas of a house, but in general the losses in the chicks in the first 4 or 5 days of life are after-effects of the management and health of the breeders or the management and hygiene in the hatchery. In the first section we will consider the commonest ailments of the chick.

Yolk-sac infection (also called 'mushy-chick' disease, omphalitis or navel infection)

This is probably the commonest of all diseases causing early mortality. The signs are clear, the chicks so affected are usually normal to start with but make no headway and die mostly from about 24–72 hours after placement in the house. Examination of the chick shows a 'blown-up' abdomen, a wet and scabby navel and a very offensive odour, which is virtually diagnostic. If the abdomen is opened it will be seen that there is copious discoloured fluid, often brown, and infections may have spread throughout the abdominal cavity. The infective agents that cause the disease are bacteria and the ubiquitous *E. coli* is frequently the main one involved.

Why does the disease occur? It may be due to a number of reasons, ranging from mismanagement of the breeder flocks or bad hygiene, to poor hatchery standards or accidents in the control of the incubator or hatchery.

It is significant that we tend to find a much higher incidence in chicks hatched towards the end of winter or in the early spring when the health and condition of the breeding flocks are usually at their lowest ebb. No treatment will save those chicks that are affected but it may be advisable to treat affected flocks since it can help to limit the spread of infection. The infected birds will release enormous numbers of potentially pathogenic organisms into the environment so the following measures may be rationally applied.

1. Increase the warmth of the house to assist the birds' resistance to infection and help to prevent huddling.
2. Have tests carried out in the laboratory to establish which organisms are involved and which treatment would be most appropriate.
3. Medicate the drinking water with a vitamin and antibiotic mixture.
4. Cull all abnormal chicks vigorously.
5. Make careful investigation of the hatchery or breeding organisation as to the likely cause. It is of great importance to do this so that the source of the disease can be located. If the breeding management is not informed of the trouble it may have no awareness of the problem and no measures will then be taken to stem its incidence.

Aspergillosis (or brooder pneumonia)

This is the most important but by no means the only disease of poultry caused by a fungus, and leads to early death. The fungus, usually *Aspergillus fumigatus*, is one that occurs widely on farms and in the countryside and can therefore quite easily contaminate hatching eggs. The fungus in natural conditions needs mouldy, damp conditions to thrive in which the moisture content is more than 20 per cent – so it can be common, for example, if breeders are kept on damp litter or there is damp and dirty material in the nests.

Hatching eggs can pick up the fungus in the nests or on the litter itself quite readily and the pathogen will then be taken through to the hatchery. If infection enters the hatchery and the fungus is not destroyed by fumigation, an almost explosive incidence can occur in the chicks and mortality in the first few days of life may vary from only a few chicks up to 50 per cent or even more on occasions. Alternatively, the chicks can themselves pick up infection from damp and mouldy litter used as their bedding.

The signs of infection are of pneumonia, the chicks gasping and struggling for breath with their mouth open. Post-mortem findings are of tiny yellowish-green nodules with a green furry extrusion in the lungs, bronchi, trachea and viscera, while the air sacs may be covered with thick yellow exudate. A laboratory will identify the fungus definitely. A certain diagnosis cannot be made by the naked eye or by the symptoms, which may be similar to other diseases.

There is no specific treatment. If outbreaks occur in chicks they act as a warning of considerable importance that there are serious errors in hygiene or management and it is vital that the areas of infection are located so that remedial steps can be taken. Control measures will include a culling of affected chicks, a more thorough disinfection of housing and equipment, removal of unsuitable litter or nesting material, and better cleaning and fumigation of hatching eggs and equipment and the hatchery. Obviously, the precise steps to be taken will depend on the place where the infection takes place.

Salmonellosis

The group of bacteria known as *Salmonella* exists world-wide and is one of the greatest causes of diseases in poultry. In many countries, including the UK, due to prolonged control measures, there are now few losses in poultry due to salmonellosis. Furthermore, it must be stressed that overriding emphasis is now attached to an attempt – which may well be achieved before long – to eradicate salmonella disease altogether from British birds because certain members of this species of bacteria are a principal cause of food poisoning in man. It will be appreciated that under intensive conditions there is an extra risk of contagion taking hold of many birds at one time, so it is highly desirable that all possible sources of infection are removed. A few areas of the world, notably Scandinavia, have been able to virtually rid themselves of salmonella infections in animals.

Types of salmonella infection
There are two forms of the salmonella species specific to poultry – *Salmonella pullorum* and *Salmonella gallinarum*. The former, perhaps the oldest of all diseases diagnosed in poultry, used to be called bacillary white diarrhoea (BWD), while *S. gallinarum* is commonly called fowl typhoid. In addition, we have those diseases in poultry caused by other salmonella and coming under the general title of salmonellosis or sometimes termed avian paratyphoid. There are many different forms – at least 200 types of salmonella have been found in poultry – but the most important are *S. typhimurium* and *S. enteriditis*, which can be virulent killers of chicks in particular.

Symptoms. The symptoms of the various forms of salmonella infection vary considerably. Mortality is extremely variable, ranging from no more than 1 or 2 per cent up to as much as 50 per cent. For example, if chicks are infected with *S. pullorum* disease via the infected dam and thereby spread through the hatchery, signs of illness will occur within a matter of hours of hatching. In cases where the infection is light and the environment and husbandry good, the losses can be modest, but early losses from salmonella infections more usually run at between 10 and 20 per cent and extend over perhaps 2 weeks. Those chicks dying early on in life usually die quickly with few symptoms but as the disease proceeds, symptoms of huddling, inappetance, constant cheeping, a swollen abdomen and white diarrhoea progressively appear. There may also be chronic cases in which numbers of chicks are stunted, scour and experience lameness due to swollen joints. It is stressed that these symptoms are much the same for all forms of salmonella infection in chicks and growing birds, and it is quite impossible from these symptoms either to distinguish which form of salmonella is present or indeed whether it is a salmonella disease at all.

In the adult, acute salmonella infection is typically that known as fowl typhoid, due to *S. gallinarum*. Signs of an attack would be when a number of birds scour with greenish-yellow, evil-smelling droppings, have a greatly increased thirst, show very pale (anaemic) head parts and there are also a number of sudden deaths. As mortality may go as high as 75 per cent with 50 per cent being common, this is a disease that is hardly likely to be missed. Post-mortem signs in the chick are not diagnostic but are at least strongly suspicious. If the bird dies at the hyper- (very) acute stage the signs are few, apart from congestion of internal organs, especially liver and lungs. In later cases where the infection is only acute or sub-acute, the liver and other internal organs show characteristic yellowy nodules and the caecal tubes often contain semi-solid yellow 'casts'. The yolk sac may likewise be filled with a pus-like 'sludge'. In the adult, the post-mortem signs in pullorum or gallinarum infections are similar, but are especially associated with the ovary in which the ovules are grossly misshapen and the contents are also abnormal. Other internal organs may be infected, including the heart, which shows inflammation of the membranes around it (pericarditis). These diagnostic symptoms in the adult are only rarely seen with the other forms of salmonella.

The control of salmonella infections

With pullorum and gallinarum infections, simple and rapid on-the-spot blood tests have been in use for many years and can detect carriers with great accuracy. These tests have been enormously successful since they enable immediate removal of the carrier birds from a flock. Thus the two diseases caused by *S. pullorum* and *S. gallinarum* have been controlled with great success in many countries, including the UK. Under these circumstances only a few isolated cases turn up from time to time detected by blood tests, and regular testing may only be necessary on the foundation breeding stock.

Unfortunately, the position with regard to other types of salmonella is entirely different and somewhat confusing. There are some 200 different serotypes that have been isolated from poultry. A few can be quite devastating in their effect, such as *Salmonella typhimurium*. Others are mild or cause no symptoms at all. In every case infection may spread to other livestock or man. It is probable, however, that the main risk is not that the poultry will infect other forms of life, but that other livestock will infect poultry.

In general, the symptoms of salmonella infection in chicks are similar to those seen in pullorum disease and indeed it is only possible to distinguish the cause by laboratory examination. Post-mortem lesions do not enable more than suspicions to be raised, although there is always the likely involvement of the liver, which is usually enlarged and congested.

Salmonella and the consumer

Salmonella has long been known as one of the most important causes of food poisoning in man. In recent years it has been recognised that *Salmonella enteriditis* is the most important serotype reported from human cases of salmonella food poisoning and it was claimed there was a clear epidemiological association of these cases with eggs, egg products and poultry meat. In 1989, the British government therefore introduced a programme of measures for the control of salmonella in eggs and poultry. The measures are aimed at reducing infections throughout the complete production chain, from the supply of feedstuffs to the production of healthy breeding stock and laying flocks.

Under the Zoonoses Order of 1989 all isolations of salmonella from samples taken from an animal or bird, or from any feedstuff must be reported to a Ministry Veterinary Officer. The Order allows Veterinary Officers to enter premises and carry out an investigation. Powers are available to declare premises infected, to prohibit the movement of animals, poultry, carcasses, products and feedstuffs in or out of the premises, except under a licence, also serving notices requiring the cleansing and disinfection of premises where salmonella is known to have been present. There are a large number of other regulations under the Zoonoses Order requiring registration and testing of breeder flocks and hatcheries and laying down procedures for slaughter or treatment if 'positives' occur. When an isolation of *S. enteriditis* is reported from a layer breeder flock, for example, a notice is served on the owner of the premises declaring it to be an infected place and prohibiting the movement of eggs, birds, food, etc. off the site except under licence. A sample of birds is then taken from each house on the premises and subjected to a detailed bacteriological examination. Investigation may also be carried out when there is evidence linking a flock to an outbreak of human food poisoning.

Feedstuffs

The Processed Animal Protein Order of 1989 requires all processors of animal protein to register with MAFF and to ensure that samples of processed animal protein consigned from their premises on any day are submitted to an approved laboratory for testing for salmonella. If a salmonella organism is isolated from the samples, no processed animal protein may be removed from the premises for incorporation into animal or poultry feedstuffs unless certain conditions specified in this Order are complied with. In addition, authorised officers carry out quarterly inspections involving the collection and bacteriological examination of samples of 20 days' production from each premises per year. There are also more rigorous licensing conditions for the importation of animal and fish protein which were introduced in 1989 under the Importation of Processed Animal Protein Order.

The effects of regulations

The effects of these regulations have been profound and there seems no reason why the poultry flock of the country cannot be rid of those forms of salmonella that cause disease in man. The cost to the poultry industry has been severe. The foundation breeding flocks have in any case been kept free of these serotypes of salmonella for a number of years and, as virtually all birds come from this stock, that would seem to indicate the end of the problem in due course. There is no doubt that British poultry products are second to none in their safety to the consumer, yet there remains a sense of unease about the matter. Our poultry may be free of these and other zoonoses but they will always be vulnerable to the introduction and re-infection from other sources, such as wildlife, over which we have no control, the whole environment around them and above all from man himself. In Sweden they have had no virulent salmonella in their birds for some time, but apparently a higher proportion of the human population suffers from salmonella infection than in the UK. Scandinavians tend to holiday in the warmer countries around the Mediterranean and elsewhere where salmonella is rife, and they become carriers. The same circumstances obviously apply to British holidaymakers. Also, animal products, including poultry, enter the UK from European Union sources in an almost unrestricted way, and several EU countries have no salmonella control programmes. Poultry products are currently entering the UK from other parts of the world where salmonella control programmes are absent. Thus, with people and animal products constantly putting our birds at risk, the UK government's policy is, at the least, worrying.

It should never be forgotten that if food is properly prepared and handled the risk of food poisoning is almost completely removed. More emphasis in this direction, together with improved codes of practice on the agricultural side would probably have been adequate and would have saved the compulsory slaughter of many millions of chickens. Politicians, vested interests and the media have been responsible for generating an emotional rather than an objective reaction and the cost has been unnecessarily high.

Respiratory disease of chicks

With the increase in the intensity and size of poultry units has come such an upsurge in the incidence of respiratory diseases that these without doubt form the most important reason for ill-health in poultry in almost all parts of the world. It is unusual nowadays to find respiratory disease in an uncomplicated form. The usual pattern is for one or more primary virus infections, acute or chronic, to be followed by secondary bacterial invaders in which strains of *E. coli* usually predominate. Preventive techniques are all-important since once respiratory disease has developed in a flock and especially the young bird, losses by mortality, or poor growth and food conversion can be so severe that it may be extremely difficult to stop a catastrophic economic loss.

The approach to preventive losses cannot be easily generalised because the types of infection vary a great deal geographically. If there is a high incidence of Newcastle disease and/or infectious bronchitis, two of the main conditions, for example, a central plank in preventative policy will be to protect the birds by vaccination. The strains of vaccine to be used and their frequency of use will be dependent on the local challenges that predominate and the parental immunity of the chicks. This parental immunity may have been derived from infection in the parent flock or from a suitable vaccination policy. As well as protection by vaccination, which will always be concerned with protecting birds from the primary viral agents, there may also be useful ways of protecting birds against the secondary bacterial infections by medication of the stock, either in the food or drinking water, with antibiotics or chemotherapeutic agents. Finally, all these measures will be supported by good husbandry methods; for example, by applying warmth, improving air flow, adding litter and changing lighting systems. We are faced once again with the salient fact that in many cases of respiratory infection it will be management rather than anything else that will influence its effect on the bird.

Infectious bronchitis (IB)

Universally, this is the most widely experienced respiratory disease and is caused by a highly contagious virus. There are a number of strains and whilst most primarily affect the respiratory system there are some varieties that also have a serious effect on the kidneys, causing what is known as the uraemic form of the disease.

Symptoms. The most noticeable sign in the young chick is a large amount of respiratory noise. Birds sneeze, gasp and shake their head and in a large flock the best way of detecting early signs is to 'look and listen'. Enter the house very quietly, or if the birds are disturbed by your entry, wait until they are still. If you listen, the 'snicking' of the birds will be clearly heard and is almost symptomatic. Early observational diagnosis is all-important because it enables immediate use of any preventive medication to be instituted. If the disease is allowed to advance unchecked the respiratory noise will get worse, there will be eye-watering, nasal discharge and increasing mortality and secondary infections which may take over, completely masking the original infection.

If the only trouble is the infectious bronchitis virus, this could be over within a week to a fortnight, but it is rare for there to be such a happy outcome. Nevertheless, if the disease is uncomplicated the effect can be mild and recovery can be complete, rather like the common cold in man. What usually happens in practice is that as soon as the birds show signs of sickness they start huddling together and this provides the ideal medium for the propagation of other infections, viral or bacterial, but often dominated by *E. coli*.

In older birds, infectious bronchitis disease can have two profound effects on the female. Infection in the immature female can prevent development of the oviduct partially or completely so that the bird will lay few, if any, eggs. In the other case, if the flock is adult and laying it will lead to a massive drop in egg production, which may partially recover, but in addition there will tend to be the production of poor quality eggs and egg shells. Eggs are often of strange shapes, the egg shells are ridged and lack pigment and the white of the egg is watery.

When layers are affected, egg production may fall to a few per cent and it *may* then recover to normal over a period of weeks. However, my own experience is that this seldom happens and this fact, taken together with the lowered egg quality, means that the loss to an egg producer can have very serious consequences. It has even worse consequences for the poultry breeder because a bronchitis infection during production can lower not only egg numbers and quality but will additionally adversely affect fertility and hatchability. All these points emphasise the importance of giving susceptible birds protection by a complete vaccination programme if there is a fair risk of a challenge with the field virus.

Post-mortem signs in chicks affected with the respiratory form will include the detection of catarrh in the trachea, congested lungs and cloudy air sacs. When the kidneys are affected, they appear considerably enlarged and white with deposits of urates. Sometimes urate deposits are seen through the body cavities. The effect on the oviduct is to reduce it in size, sometimes so much so that it is almost absent, while with the mature bird the misshapen ova are diagnostic.

Diagnosis. The symptoms of infectious bronchitis after an incubation period of usually 1–4 days appear to be so reasonably straightforward that they would allow clinical diagnosis to be effected without laboratory tests, but because the occurrence of the disease is rarely without other intruders, it is often necessary to have samples dealt with at the laboratory to be certain. For example, as shall be seen in the ensuing sections, the milder forms of Newcastle disease or mycoplasmosis can produce rather similar symptoms. In any case, once the secondaries have come up to have their damaging effects, the diagnostic signs have all been very well masked. Thus plenty of use is made of the various tests, either by virus isolation or by specific antibodies in the sera. The great advantage of having a positive diagnosis done is that while it is most likely that the result will not be in time to influence the treatment to be used in the flock in question, it may be possible to plan or modify future control measures in the light of this information.

Control. Details of the approach to the control of the disease are given at the end of the section on Newcastle disease because it is best to consider these two rather similar diseases together.

Newcastle disease (ND)
Just like infectious bronchitis, Newcastle disease tends to occur throughout the world wherever there are large poultry populations. While the first outbreak that was reported and described occurred in Newcastle, England in 1927,

this came as an importation of the most virulent form of the disease, which occurred in the Far East. The first outbreaks that occurred in those days were nearly all extremely virulent and killed off virtually all affected and in-contact birds. Since that time, various other forms of the disease have occurred, many being much milder in extent and others somewhere between the two extremes. At the time of writing the most virulent cases appear to occur in the warmer countries and the milder cases in the more temperate climates. The last serious outbreak in the UK started in Essex as long ago as 1970 but the so-called 'Essex 70' strain which could cause almost 100 per cent mortality has now disappeared from the British Isles. There have been sporadic outbreaks of moderately pathogenic forms, the last one at the beginning of 1998 in Ireland and England.

Any outbreak is countered by the slaughter of all infected flocks and any possible contacts that could be incubating the disease. Vaccination might be used under official direction in a ring around an infected area to prevent the infection escaping from a small focal point.

Symptoms. The incubation period of ND is usually 2–7 days but may be prolonged up to 3 weeks. Normally the first signs in a flock are an unusual lassitude and indifference to food and water throughout the flock. This complete lack of the normal reactions of lively birds is quite symptomatic. There may be signs of respiratory distress, some birds apparently struggling for breath, with weird high pitched 'cries' issuing forth in isolated cases, a symptom which does not seem to occur with any other diseases. The nervous signs show up as a drooping of either one or both wings, lack of co-ordination, falling over and paddling of the legs and twitching and twisting of the neck muscles.

If the three main groups of symptoms are found in a flock then the presence of ND would be fairly certain, but a diagnostic check should always be made and in any case it is unlikely that the pattern would be quite so logically presented as may have been implied.

Only some of the symptoms might be seen. Confusion can occur with several other diseases and also, if some protection has been afforded by parental immunity or partial vaccination, the end picture would be a very different one. For example, in layers the only effect might be a drop in the egg production and egg quality, without a subsequent regain to normality. It will already be apparent that confusion with infectious bronchitis could be very easy and there may be many more diseases that could be confused with it.

Post-mortem signs. Some or all of the following signs may be seen: the respiratory tract is usually inflamed, the air sacs are cloudy and there are small haemorrhages, known as 'petechiae' on the heart and proventriculus (especially).

There is often a great deal of caseous (dried, pus-like) material in the trachea and bronchi and haemorrhages can be seen on the mucous membranes of the respiratory system.

Diagnosis. Clinical symptoms as described, together with the most prominent post-mortem signs as have been indicated, may be sufficient to be almost sure but it is always necessary to have laboratory tests done. This may be done by virus isolation and/or serological testing; the tests will be able to identify the virulence of the particular strain of the virus.

Control measures. If we start with the chick, in most cases where the disease is prevalent, it will be necessary to vaccinate all parent flocks very thoroughly. It is then likely that the chicks will be hatched with a good immunity. There may not seem very much point in an immediate vaccination and while this is not entirely true there are good practical reasons in large flocks to give some protection almost as soon after hatching as possible. One reason is that in large houses of many thousands of birds there will almost certainly be some chicks that do not have an immunity. Thus, an early vaccination will protect them. Furthermore, if an early vaccination is given, it has been found that later vaccination will cause less stress. The problem of stress cannot be exaggerated. The vaccines now used on chicks by water or spray administration are very effective but they are live and mildly virulent. Properly used they will cause little or no harmful effects but if incorrectly or carelessly used they are quite capable of causing a severe reaction which may be followed by secondary infections that can be almost as bad as the disease.

Protection of the birds against Newcastle disease and infectious bronchitis

For Newcastle disease there are three widely used vaccines, two being live vaccines (Hitchner B_1 and La Sota) and one an inactivated oil-based vaccine. The first two are administered by spray, drinking water, or occasionally eye-drop, while the oil-based vaccine is given by intra-muscular injection. Hitchner B_1 is a safe, 'gentle' vaccine that can be given by mass techniques such as a spray and provides instant protection but only for a few weeks. La Sota is a little more stressful but is still mild and will protect for up to 12 weeks in the more mature bird. There are also 'clone' vaccines with extremely mild effects but better protection. The oil-based vaccine by injection is most frequently used in the older bird – commonly at point of lay, and will protect for a laying season but does not give immediate protection. Nevertheless, it seems that within this 'armoury' of vaccines the protection needed for any set of circumstances can usually be found, although in countries where the most virulent forms of Newcastle disease are present, it is usual to have some of the more powerful vaccines available, such as the Komarov. These have the disadvantage that they cause very considerable stress on the birds, hence most countries will not license their use.

There are several commonly used live vaccines to protect birds against infectious bronchitis. There are the relatively mild Massachusetts type H-120 which is used early in life and gives immediate and limited protection, and the H-52 which gives a much longer protection. There are also further live vaccines available to protect against a number of variant infectious bronchitis viruses. It must be emphasised that full protection must be provided at all stages during development, not only to ensure that the birds throw off any challenge that might cause respiratory disease, but also because of the danger that if a potential layer or breeder contracts the disease during its development the reproductive organs can be so damaged that egg production will be profoundly affected. Alternatively, an inactivated oil-based vaccine may be given to protect adult birds.

In Table 11.1 are given certain programmes of protection which can be used either as a general routine protection where indicated, or for special emergencies or where there are severe challenges. It is as well to emphasise that even in the presence of Newcastle disease it is possible to spray birds with a large droplet (about 50 μm in size) and this may arrest the course of the disease on the site since the vaccine particles have a 'blocking' effect by giving localised protection via the cells of the respiratory mucous membranes. In this connection it is well to stress the virtues of the large particle sprayer, such as the Turbair illustrated, compared with the small particle aerosol which it is best *not* to use. The latter penetrates deeply into the respiratory system and can cause a serious reaction. A method of using infectious bronchitis and Newcastle disease vaccines at day-old, if desired in the hatchery, has been developed by using a sufficiently large particle spray with considerable success, as it gives a minimum of reaction and a maximum of protection.

Mycoplasma infection (CRD)

Mycoplasma are a group of organisms that cause a great deal of disease in the animal population. They are not dissimilar to, but are still quite distinct from bacteria, being smaller and free living, which distinguishes them from viruses.

In livestock they are mostly associated with respiratory diseases and the poultry disease known as 'chronic respiratory disease' (CRD) is primarily caused by *Mycoplasma gallisepticum*. The usual signs of the disease in a flock are sneezing, snicking and coughing, inflamed and running eyes and swelling of the sinuses of the face. The lesions to be seen in the bird are likely to be confined to the respiratory tract and will consist of varying degrees of inflammation and exudates in the tract linings and the air sac. The disease in itself can cause

Table 11.1 Newcastle disease and infectious bronchitis vaccination by the use of a large particle spray, or via drinking water or by injection[a]

Age	Method	Vaccine		Remarks
		Broilers	Breeders/layers	
1–4 days General sensitising dose	Spray	B$_1$ & H-120	B$_1$ & H-120	Helps to reduce stress from subsequent vaccination
Primary vaccination 12–14 days	Spray	B$_1$ & H-120	B$_1$	No necessity to use both if risk is small
Secondary vaccination 22–28 days	Spray	B$_1$ or La Sota	B$_1$ or La Sota	No necessity to use both if risk is small
35–42 days	Spray	B$_1$ or La Sota	B$_1$ or La Sota	Final vaccination for broilers; unnecessary if low risk
10 weeks	Spray La Sota		La Sota or inactivated and H-52	
Just before point of lay	Spray or injection		La Sota or inactivated	Inactivated oil-based vaccines recommended for this application; La Sota live vaccine will give a much shorter immunity and necessitates re-vaccination during lay

Boosting during lay – La Sota needs re-vaccinating after 5 months; no re-vaccination with inactivated.
[a]La Sota vaccine is not currently allowed in the UK.

Note: (1) Spray vaccination is generally more effective than application by drinking water, provided it is correctly applied. Spray vaccination can increase the problem of coli-septicaemia, and in these flocks drinking water application may be used as an alternative.

(2) Spray vaccination works in two ways: it induces a rapid rise in and also gives a useful measure of protection on respiratory surfaces themselves, known as a 'local block'.

(3) Combined vaccines of IB + ND + TRT + Gumboro are frequently used as inactivated injections in layers of breeder replacements.

(4) Ma5 and Clone 30 can replace B$_1$ and H-120 in sprays or water.

some mortality and loss of productivity but it is very often a precursor to the other respiratory diseases. It is more serious in its effects on the young bird than the older one.

Control. Mycoplasmosis is a less contagious and less acutely virulent disease then the worst forms of Newcastle disease or infectious bronchitis. There is no vaccine available to prevent it but nevertheless it may be controlled very effectively in several ways. The most satisfactory way is to build up an entire breeding enterprise that is free of disease by blood testing and elimination of infected birds. There are good serological tests and this procedure has been so successful that most breeding stock in the UK and USA and Western Europe are now largely free of *M. gallisepticum* infection. There are also several antibiotics that will successfully control the disease so these may be used in conjunction with a blood testing programme.

Because the organisms can be transmitted from hen to chick via the egg, it is also recommended to treat the hatching eggs in infected breeder flocks by dipping them in suitable solutions containing anti-mycoplasmal drugs.

A related mycoplasma, *M. synoviae*, is also a widespread cause of disease. While it is primarily a cause of lameness due to the inflammation it causes in leg joints, it also retards growth and causes respiratory infections. Control measures are similar to those for *M. gallisepticum.*

Infectious laryngotracheitis (ILT)

Infectious laryngotracheitis (or ILT, as it is more popularly termed for obvious reasons!) is a highly virulent viral disease that is world-wide in incidence but is confined to certain areas. Symptoms are usually of an extremely serious respiratory involvement with great distress exhibited by the birds as they struggle for breath, accompanied by coughing and rattling and often with the birds depositing bloody mucous. There may also be less acute forms of the disease which are less severe but otherwise similar. Post-mortem examination of birds with ILT shows severe inflammation of the larynx and trachea with bloody, cheesy 'clots' virtually filling the trachea. The virus that causes ILT does not affect any other organs and the birds die of asphyxiation.

Diagnosis can be made with a considerable degree of certainty from the symptoms, post-mortem picture and history, but because the signs are not always as clear as has been suggested and there may well be other complicating factors, it is advisable to have a laboratory 'check' on specimens and if necessary to seek virus isolations or serological tests.

Treatment and prevention. There is no drug available that will affect the viruses of ILT and the only effect of treatment with antibiotics and vitamin supplements will be to assist the birds' resistance to secondary infections. There are good vaccines available to prevent the disease. Recovered birds may remain as carriers of the infection for the rest of their lives. Thus, in an 'elimination' programme it is best to start by depopulating the entire site and then follow through with a most rigorous cleaning and disinfection programme. This is also one case at least where it would be advisable to leave the premises empty for a few weeks after the disinfection programme has been completed.

Infectious coryza (roup)

A bacterium, *Haemophilus gallinarum,* can cause a disease in poultry which is rather akin to the common cold in man. The symptoms are acute, lead to general inflammation, swelling and discharges around and from the eyes and the nose. It does not appear to be a very serious problem nowadays in intensive units but vaccines are made which are effective in preventing it. Treatment of the condition is to use antibiotics to which the organism is found to be sensitive after suitable tests.

Gumboro disease (infectious bursal disease)

This is an extremely important infection in most areas of the world, first reported in 1962 in the village of Gumboro in the USA and very soon afterwards appearing in the UK and Western Europe. The symptoms of the disease are rather indefinite but generally first show as an acute infection of young chicks, mostly broilers, of sudden onset. There is a quick peak of mortality, followed by a return to normality, but which leaves a substantial number of birds stunted in their growth and very unproductive. Affected chicks show anorexia, depression, huddling, ruffled feathers, vent pecking, diarrhoea, trembling and lack of co-ordination. The most significant post-mortem sign is an extreme inflammation of the bursa of Fabricius (see Figure 3.1), which will be greatly enlarged, and oedematous. Haemorrhages may be seen here and in the muscles of the body and the kidneys may be swollen, pale and contain urate deposits.

While the disease may not cause a high mortality, usually in the region of 5 per cent, the other effects of the disease must not be underestimated. The stunting in some of the survivors has already been stressed, but even more serious is the fact that the virus, by adversely affecting the bursa of Fabricius, causes profound damage to the whole immunological system of the chicken. The chick may suffer from other diseases in consequence, especially as it may now be unable to get proper protection from vaccines. In many ways, it is this last effect which is the most serious one and will be considered further in this chapter.

Some 10 years ago a more virulent form of Gumboro disease became prevalent in various parts of the world and has now spread to virtually all of the larger poultry growing areas. The worst effects have been in broilers, especially cockerels, and mortality can reach 40 per cent at least if the birds are unprotected. Dealing with Gumboro disease involves three procedures. The first is hygiene to the highest standard, to minimise or at least delay the likely challenge on succeeding crops. The virus causing Gumboro disease is an extremely persistent one and it is unlikely to be completely eliminated by cleaning and disinfection. Second, protection is given to the chicks by the use of a live vaccine administered by spray or in the drinking water. A wide range of vaccines of varying strengths are available; the choice will be dependent on the degree of the local challenge expected, but at its worst it may be necessary to give mild vaccines to a broiler flock two or three times. This is not necessary with the 'hotter strains' of vaccines now available. There are also very effective inactivated vaccines for use in breeders so that they pass on a strong passive immunity to the chicks that should protect them up to 4 weeks of age. Unfortunately, the more virulent form of the virus breaks through the maternal immunity much earlier than this so the chicks may have to be protected almost from day-old.

The infectious stunting syndrome (malabsorption syndrome or runting and stunting syndrome)

A new condition appeared in several countries of the world several years ago affecting chiefly broilers and known as the infectious stunting or malabsorption syndrome. This disease is chararacterised by severe stunting of chicks arising very soon after they go into the broiler house – it is usually first noticeable at about 10 days old. Sometimes the condition is called 'helicopter disease' because feathering is very bad and certain of the wing feathers protrude horizontally from the bird. The syndrome may affect anything from 5 to 40 per cent of the flock and by the killing age of about 50 days the affected birds will weigh about half their normal weight. Deaths are relatively few; a characteristic post-mortem sign in affected birds is a grossly atrophied pancreas, and it is assumed that the agent causing this infection has a specific effect on this organ so that the digestion and absorption of food is badly affected. Thus, afflicted birds grow very slowly, with an extremely poor food conversion efficiency.

It is known to be a highly contagious infection, certainly viral in origin, but the agents have not all been positively identified. There is no very useful treatment for the affected birds; the sooner they are culled the better, but in flocks under risk the day-old chicks may be given preventive broad-spectrum antibiotic treatment and soluble vitamin supplementation.

To eliminate infection from the site, apply the most rigorous cleaning and disinfection programme and even in earth-floored houses the disease can be eliminated. It is another example of the beneficial effects of a depopulation and disinfection programme between batches. In many cases it seems that broiler groups that practise good hygiene stay almost clear of the disease, although side-by-side in the same area, broiler companies with bad hygiene procedures suffer badly.

Clostridial diseases

There are a significant number of clostridial bacteria capable of causing disease on the poultry farm. Clostridial bacteria are a large group which are capable of 'building up' as a problem, if the site is kept unhygienically, is overstocked, or is badly constructed. Diseases caused by clostridia are malignant oedema (or gangrenous dermatitis), necrotic enteritis and botulism. Clostridial organisms may also be found in association with many other diseases as 'secondaries', for example in yolk-sac infection. There is also strong evidence that the weakening of the birds' immunity by Gumboro disease may be the forerunner to certain of these, especially malignant oedema.

Malignant oedema

Malignant oedema (or gangrenous dermatitis) is an especially objectionable, distressing and serious disease of broilers, caused by *Clostridium septicum*, which has tended to become more common. It usually occurs towards the end of the growing cycle and may cause a massive mortality – even up to 50 per cent. The effect is to cause gangrene of the muscle and of the skin so that the birds in a sense 'fall apart' while still alive.

It is often stated and believed that malignant oedema is associated with bad hygienic practices, the re-use of old litter for example, and also overstocking and bad environmental conditions. There is probably a measure of truth in this but the disease can certainly occur without any of these being obvious and the author has seen its devastating effects in flocks which are kept impeccably. What is known, however, is that it often happens after birds have had their immunity suppressed with diseases, such as Gumboro disease, or where other debilitating diseases such as inclusion body hepatitis (see next page) have occurred. Also, it should be noted that while *Clostridium septicum* may be a main infective agent with malignant oedema, it is by no means the only one involved and *Staphylococcus aureus* can be the predominant bacteria. Thus, while penicillin-G is the antibiotic of choice to deal with the infection where clostridial organisms are involved, it may be less effective against staphylococcus. It is also important where outbreaks occur to consider carefully the programme for controlling Gumboro disease because outbreaks of this condition so often precede the attacks of malignant oedema.

Necrotic enteritis

This is also a disease that is more usually found in broilers than in other types of chicken, although not exclusively so. The clostridium involved is *Cl. perfringens* and the condition can lead to a mortality of 5–10 per cent. Lesions are confined to the small intestine, which is grossly inflamed and distended.

The clostridial disease, like others, has often been found in poultry houses with earth or chalk floors where the disease organisms can 'build up' in certain areas which are probably inadequately cleaned or disinfected. Fortunately, earth floors are becoming more of a rarity but where they are used it is worthy of emphasis that they can still be disinfected reasonably adequately with the modern disinfecting materials available (see Chapter 8). Preventive or curative procedure is effective using appropriate penicillin preparations.

A very recent cause of outbreaks of necrotic enteritis has been associated with the use of 'shuttle' *Coccidiostat coccidiosis* control programmes in broilers. These generally rely on a chemical coccidiostat until about 3–4 weeks, followed by an ionophore. In addition, the broiler grower has lost the use of some good growth promoters that suppressed the clostridia.

When such an occurrence takes place it will almost always demand a review of the coccidiosis control programme and a change in the medicines used.

Botulism

This is another disease of poultry caused by a clostridium (*Cl. botulinum*) which has occurred predominantly in broilers and can cause heavy mortality. There have been cases of 20 per cent losses in birds near the killing age of 45 days. The course of this disease is rather different from other clostridia insofar as the organisms multiply in the gut, releasing a toxin that causes paralysis of the muscles, especially of the head to neck.

Fortunately, it is relatively uncommon. The type of clostridium causing botulism in chickens is *not* the same as that causing the disease in man. There is no treatment for poultry suffering from this condition but cases are usually associated with dirty sites that are badly managed.

Inclusion body hepatitis (IBH)

IBH is a relative newcomer to the poultry field, also associated mainly with broiler chickens. It occurs generally in the age range 30–50 days. It has no special symptoms except that in a flock that is probably growing very well and apparently in the best of health, a sudden heavy mortality takes place which may give a loss of up to 10 per cent. Post-mortem signs are usually confined to the liver and kidneys, the former being much enlarged and containing many haemorrhages, while the kidneys are also enlarged with haemorrhages throughout. A laboratory examination should be made to confirm the presence of this disease, which is apparently caused by a virus.

Fatty liver kidney syndrome (FLKS)

This is an interesting and nowadays relatively uncommon disease of poultry of about 7–35 days old. The symptoms are indefinite – usually there is a rather higher mortality than there should be, and a few birds will be seen lying face downwards and apparently paralysed. Post-mortem examination of the affected birds shows a pale, swollen liver with haemorrhages, the heart also pale and the kidneys swollen and usually inflamed. It should be noted that it is usually the best birds that are affected by this condition and it is associated with excessive levels of fat deposition.

Cause. It has now been established that FLKS is a disease induced by feeding high levels of wheat with lower than normal levels of protein so that the ratio between carbohydrate and protein is too wide (see Chapter 4). It has also been confirmed that if diets containing these incorrect levels are fed, then supplementation of the diet to give levels of biotin, as detailed in Chapter 3, will prevent FLKS. Now that this fact is known, the condition is rather uncommon but it does occur from time to time, due, for example, to omissions by the compounders of the added biotin.

Coccidiosis

Coccidiosis in undoubtedly the most important parasitic disease of poultry and yet, because of the successful development of drugs and vaccines to prevent and treat the condition, it is no longer a disease to be feared. Nevertheless, because it is always a potential threat which can cause serious loss, it is essential that the poultryman knows when to suspect it and what to do in an emergency. He should also be aware of the range of drugs and vaccines available and how they may be used effectively.

Coccidiosis of poultry is caused by protozoa (single-celled parasites) which live in the lining (epithelium) of the intestine. Those affecting poultry are of the species Eimeria. The life cycle of the various species in poultry is as follows. There is a massive multiplication of the coccidia (known as schizogony) and sexual multiplication (known as gametogony) within the bird. Then a stage of development takes place outside the host in which the eggs that are shed in sexual development reach a stage when they can infect other birds, although they do not multiply. These are known as oocysts.

There are nine strains of Eimeria species that can cause diseases of the intestines in poultry. Each species causes rather different symptoms due to the Eimeria parasites of each strain having different favoured sites in the intestine. For example, the most common ones are *E. tenella*, which affects only the caecal tubes and *E. necatrix*, which affects mainly the middle and lower intestine.

Symptoms. The overall symptoms may be one or more of the following: bloody droppings, high mortality, general droopiness, emaciation, a marked drop in feed consumption, diarrhoea and egg production drop in layers. Table 11.2 summarises the difference between the main species. These details show that there are certain differences in symptoms, but a skilled diagnosis is often required for any certainty and can be made from a detailed examination of the post-mortem material in a veterinary laboratory. It is desirable that good use is made of these skills since the type of coccidia found will give guidance on the reason for the infection, how to prevent it and how to treat it.

Outbreaks of coccidiosis may be treated successfully with a range of medicines, such as sulphonamides or combinations of sulphonamides and pyrimidines or amprolium, all given in the drinking water.

A wide range of coccidiostats is used to prevent the disease during the growing period. A selection of these is set out in Table 11.3. Changes of medicines are appropriate by careful planning to prevent resistance developing. Certain coccidiostats must be withdrawn a specified number of days before birds are slaughtered to ensure that there are no residues in the carcass. Because of this, it may be advantageous to use two anti-coccidial agents, even in the short life of the broiler, as it is risky to try and dispense with any prevention during the last 10 days or so of growth. Replacement birds should not be given an agent that completely destroys the parasites, since no immunity then develops. It may be surmised, and correctly, that the choice, dose and programme for the use of these highly important agents demands a skilled knowledge of the medicines and the particular circumstances of their use. In addition to the medicines, there are now vaccines available that give very effective protection and are currently used for replacement birds. Vaccines are now also available for use in broilers.

Coccidial immunity

It is especially important with the disease of coccidiosis to know how immunity develops. If birds are to achieve immunity they must ingest a sufficient

Table 11.2 Coccidiosis in poultry

Species	Age group most often affected[a]	Key symptoms	Post-mortem signs
E. tenella	4–8 weeks; cases reported as early as 7–14 days	Bloody droppings; marked drop in feed consumption; emaciation; high rate of mortality; lethargy very noticeable	Caeca filled with blood; cheesy caecal core streaked with blood
E. necatrix	6 weeks to 4 months; cases as early as 2 weeks; variable mortality	Feed consumption drops; birds droopy; loss of weight; drop in egg production	Middle of intestine involved (longer section in severe infections); small, white spots interspersed with bright or dull-red spots of variable size on unopened gut wall; wall thickened (sausage-like swelling up to twice normal size); haemorrhage into intestines; caecal contents may be tinged with blood
E. acervulina		Loss of appetite; drop in egg production; loss of weight; some diarrhoea; chronic condition in layers	Upper half of intestine affected; numerous, grey-white streaks on gut wall visible
E. praevox		Some diarrhoea; relatively harmless; no deaths	Upper third of small intestine; some degree of inflammation
E. mitis		Diarrhoea principal symptom; no mortality	Entire small intestine may be affected; slight degree of inflammation
E. brunetti	May affect young or old birds	Diarrhoea; emaciation; some mortality in serious outbreaks	Lower half of intestine affected; rectum, caeca and cloaca inflamed and thickened; entire mucosa may slough in severe outbreak
E. maxima		Diarrhoea; droppings may be flecked with blood; loss of appetite; emaciation; some death	Dilation and thickening of lower half of intestine; gut filled with pink mucus or greyish-brown exudate
E. hagani	Older birds usually affected	Some diarrhoea; relatively harmless; no deaths	Upper half of small intestine; small, round haemorrhagic spots visible through serosa in duodenum
E. mivati	May affect young or old birds	Unthriftness; severe infections cause marked morbidity; drop in egg production	Early stages in anterior third of small intestine Later in lower small intestine, caeca and rectum Rounded lesions congestion and white opacities, blood-tinged to watery faeces

[a]Birds of any age may be affected.

number of oocysts, then go through several life cycles and multiply. Following exposure with a sufficient number of oocysts the bird will then become resistant to the disease. Immunity must be established for each individual species of coccidia because there is no cross immunity, thus birds can become immune to one species of coccidia yet still be vulnerable to others. Also, it is noteworthy that immunity is not permanent. It can be lost if the environment of the bird does not provide a sufficient level of re-exposure. In certain tests loss of immunity was demonstrated within as short a period as 10 weeks.

Two principles are used to achieve the gradual production of immunity as a means of controlling coccidiosis. The first is by the use of medicines at low level to reduce the severity of natural exposure and the second deliberate feeding of the litter with coccidia to provide a controlled exposure. It is much safer and more reliable to use anti-coccidial medicines. With both of these methods it is possible to have an inadequate exposure with a resultant deficiency in immunity, or an excessive exposure leading to losses from the disease.

The most common technique to control coccidiosis is to give continuous preventive medication for a defined period with one of the anti-coccidial medicines in the food. All broiler chicken are given this treatment and so are some replacement breeding and egg production stock, although the use of vaccine now dominates this field. Adult birds are usually not given preventive medication since they should have achieved immunity by then.

Withdrawal of coccidiostats
In practical terms, the difficulty of dealing with the use and withdrawal of coccidiostats in young rearing birds must be stressed, as opposed to using the vaccine. The chicks will usually be put on a coccidiostat from hatching and this is likely to both control the disease and allow the chicks to build up an immunity, so that by the time the drug is taken off, say, between 12 and 16 weeks of age, a satisfactory level of immunity has developed and the birds can safely withstand any subsequent challenge. Birds must be very diligently watched after the withdrawal period because they may suffer from an outbreak of the clinical disease if the challenge is too great and will need treatment with one of the medicines or medicine combinations mentioned earlier. For example, damp, wet litter following a period of satisfactory dry conditions might favour a sudden outburst of coccidial activity.

Factors affecting infectivity
An initial factor affecting the course of the disease is the viability of the oocysts and their survival on the ground. Infected birds excrete enormous numbers of oocysts in their droppings in the fresh (unsporulated) stage. The oocysts are not capable of infecting birds until a further stage of development has taken

place. If conditions are just right for sporulation it will take place within two days. Such conditions are warmth (25–35°C) with a high moisture content, which are not uncommon in the poultry field. However, if the environment is unfavourable, sporulation may take a long time or not take place at all; for example, at temperatures below 10°C, or very dry conditions. If the temperature is very high (for example, 45–50°C for a day or 56°C for an hour) the oocysts will be destroyed.

Once the oocysts have sporulated they are quite resistant to low temperatures (but not a hard frost) and are relatively resistant to dry conditions, and many forms of disinfectants that would kill viruses or bacteria. They are, however, killed by temperatures above 56°C and by ammonia and methylbromide gases.

In practical terms, this means that oocysts can even survive outside the birds on the ground for up to 2 years. However, on deep litter the combination of dryness, ammonia production and bacterial decomposition results in the destruction of oocysts within about 2 weeks of being voided. Information on the appropriate use of disinfectants is given in Chapter 8.

Blackhead (histomoniasis)

Blackhead is another disease caused by a protozoa parasite called *Histomonas meleagridis*. While it is primarily a disease of turkeys, it may also affect young chickens in a relatively mild form. The symptoms include watery, yellowish diarrhoea, lethargy, weakness and loss of appetite. Post-mortem examination shows a marked inflammation, usually with cheesy cores in the lumen of the caeca; on the liver a number of circular yellowish-green depressions or ulcers about 12 mm in diameter may be observed.

There are a number of medicines that may be used for prevention or cure of blackhead, such as Emtryl (Merial) and Salfuride (Fort Dodge). The occurrence of blackhead in chickens indicates a need to improve hygiene and eliminate intestinal worms since their eggs may carry the blackhead parasites.

Viral arthritis (tenosynovitis)

A widespread form of viral arthritis is quite common in broiler chickens from about 4 weeks onwards. The signs are of serious lameness in the birds coupled with poor growth rates and bad food conversion. In the affected birds the flexor tendon sheaths running along the posterior of the tarsometatarsal bones are visibly swollen, giving the shanks a very enlarged appearance. The sheaths of the gastrocnemius tendons themselves may frequently rupture. At a post-mortem examination the sheaths can be seen to be oedematous, looking almost like gelatine in appearance. There is usually no pus in the inflamed tissues and the remainder of the bird appears completely normal.

It is often possible to make a diagnosis on the basis of the clinical signs but confirmation depends upon virus isolation and identification. There seems little doubt that the virus causing this condition is widely spread in the world's poultry industries but only certain broiler flocks are without maternal immunity and are challenged. Thus the practical incidence of the disease is quite limited. There is no cure for the condition, but when flocks are affected the administration of an antibiotic with a wide spectrum of activity plus soluble vitamin preparations is a justified veterinary procedure in order to limit the effect of the disease, guard against secondaries, such as staphylococci and clostridia, and help to overcome the effects of inappetence and poor growth. Recent experience has shown the benefits of preventing the disease with a course of 'Reo' vaccines.

Epidemic tremor (infectious avian encephalomyelitis; IAE)

The condition of epidemic tremor is caused by a specific virus of chicken leading to nervous signs and symptoms in young birds. While birds of all ages can be infected, it is only in birds up to about 8 weeks of age that the characteristic nervous signs are normally seen. In laying birds an attack causes a drop in egg production of about 10 per cent which is soon over, but a drop in hatchability also occurs.

The signs that would lead to suspicion of this disease are confined to the nervous system. Chicks show inco-ordinate movements, falling, collapsing, then becoming prostrate and finally dying. If the chick is picked up and rested in the palm of the hand the tremors of the muscle may be felt, which are quite characteristic of the disease. Usually about 10–15 per cent of the flock are affected and most of them die, although a few do make a complete recovery. A definite diagnosis is made on microscopic examination of the brain and central nervous system where specific diagnostic changes take place.

Route of infection. The virus infects chicks in two ways. The first route is from the dam to the chick via the ovaries. After hatching the virus can enter by the mouth or respiratory system. If chicks are infected via the ovary, they contract the disease within about 7 days of hatching. If the chicks are infected by the oral route, they will become diseased from about 3 weeks onwards.

Control. Fortunately, excellent live vaccines are now available to control epidemic tremor. The procedure undertaken is to vaccinate breeders to protect them against falls in egg production and hatchability and also to prevent the transfer of infection to their chicks. Vaccination is given between 10 and 16 weeks of age. Provided it is done within this period, protection should be satisfactory for the rest of the life.

Mycotoxicosis

It is worth noting that chicks of all ages may be affected with forms of the disease known as mycotoxicosis. This is really a group of diseases that arise from toxins released by moulds found chiefly in certain feedstuffs or in the litter of poultry houses. Symptoms are usually indefinite, but there may be a number of birds off-colour, obviously sick, droopy, eating and drinking little or nothing and several dying. Post-mortem signs are mostly confined to the liver which may be congested in acute cases, or in chronic cases pale, or yellowish-brown in colour and hard. Confirmation of the involvement of a mycotoxin present requires detailed microscopic examination of the liver, and of the feed the birds have been receiving. There is no specific treatment but the administration of vitamins is warranted, especially B vitamins in the water, in an attempt to reduce some of the effects of the toxins. A number of chemicals are currently available for the treatment of either the food or the litter and housing.

Marek's disease and leucosis

Both Marek's disease and lymphoid leucosis are very important conditions of the chick which cause neoplasms (tumours) by two groups of viruses. Marek's disease is caused by a strongly cell-associated herpes virus, while leucosis is caused by some of the so-called RNA tumour virus group of oncornaviruses. The major manifestation in both diseases is lymphoid neoplasia, but in other respects the two conditions differ widely.

Marek's disease

Marek's disease was probably the most common of all poultry diseases before the relatively recent introduction of vaccines which has enabled its very successful control. It is a disease that causes proliferation of the lymphoid tissue, affecting most organs and tissues but with a special predilection for the peripheral nerves. It affects chickens most commonly between 12 and 24 weeks of age, although it does occur occasionally in chickens from 6 weeks of age and sometimes, but rarely in birds older than 24 weeks. The incubation period may vary from as little as 3 weeks to several months. One form of Marek's disease, known as *acute Marek's*, produces a very high mortality; up to 30 per cent is quite common and on occasions even up to 80 per cent. The disease may proceed in two ways: there may be a quick peak of mortality, rapidly falling away to almost nothing, all in a period of only a week or two, or alternatively, it may reach a peak quite quickly and then continue without much change for months. Only a proportion of birds may show nervous signs of paralysis.

The alternative and until more recent times, the more common form is that known as the 'classical' Marek's disease. In this, mortality is usually much less, rarely exceeding 10–15 per cent. In some cases, mortality continues only for a few weeks and in others it may go on for many months. The symptoms differ widely depending on which nerves are affected. Most often there is a progressive paralysis of the wings and legs. Badly affected birds cannot stand and a characteristic situation is to find birds lying on their sides with one leg stretched forward and the other held behind. In other cases the neck may be twisted, the respiratory system may be involved, or even the intestines.

On post-mortem examination, most typical signs with acute Marek's are diffuse lymphomatous enlargement of one or more organs or tissues, most often liver, gonads, spleen, kidneys, lungs, proventriculus and heart. Sometimes the lymphomas also arise in the skin associated with feather follicles and also in the skeletal muscles. In younger birds the liver enlargement is usually moderate in extent but in adults the greatly enlarged liver may appear identical to that in lymphoid leucosis. A new strain known as the 'J' strain has recently occurred in broiler parents and broilers world-wide, and has caused serious losses.

Control. There is no treatment for Marek's disease. Control depends on the rearing of young stock in isolation from older birds, the use of genetically resistant stock wherever possible, and above all else, by vaccination. There are several types of vaccine – these being modified field strains of Marek's disease virus or a turkey herpes virus, the latter being a virus antigenically closely related to the Marek's disease virus, which is present in most turkey flocks. It is not pathogenic for turkeys or chicks and can be used very successfully for vaccination. A good procedure to give protection is to use the so-called Rispens vaccine at day-old followed by the turkey herpes vaccine at 2–3 weeks.

There are two forms of the vaccines produced. In one form, the vaccine is used in association with the cells, and in the other the vaccines are freeze-dried. There is no evidence as to which is definitely the best and both can be recommended. The freeze-dried vaccine, which can be kept in an ordinary refrigerator, is much easier to store and handle than the cell-associated form, which must be kept in liquid nitrogen containers at −100°C. However, some poultrymen consider the immunity derived from the cell-associated form is better, perhaps because rather greater care must be taken in its handling.

The vaccines are used at day-old and are most conveniently given at the hatchery. Within a week a reasonable level of protection is obtained and this lasts a lifetime. There have been some unfortunate 'breakdowns' in properly vaccinated flocks. There is no evidence that this is due to any fault in the existing advice or techniques, but it is a warning that all the above points must be taken care of; viz. isolation of chicks, good hygiene at all stages, correct storage of vaccine, correct usage and administration of vaccine. Such has been the concern in the poultry industry about the 'breakdowns', that some organisations are now advising a second vaccination at about 2 weeks of age.

Leucosis

There are several different forms of avian leucosis. The most common is lymphoid leucosis, in which there is usually an enlargement of the liver, which is so grossly overgrown that it extends the full length of the abdominal cavity, while tumours may also affect any other organs of the body, the commonest sites being the spleen, kidney and bursa of Fabricius. Another type is erythroid leucosis, which causes very serious anaemia due to the proliferation of excessive numbers of immature red blood cells. The liver, spleen and bone marrow become cherry red in this form. In contrast, in myeloid leucosis there is tumour formation in the liver and spleen, the liver often assuming the appearance of morocco leather and a granular texture. This is due to the presence of a large number of discrete and nodular tumours of a chalky or cheesy consistency. The lesions are all caused by a group of closely related RNA tumour viruses. Virus strains produce predominantly one form of leucosis but many will also produce lymphoid leucosis. The viruses can be identified by the presence of a group of specific antigens using the so-called Cofal test.

The course of the disease. Most commercial poultry have a certain degree of infection with some groups of the leucosis viruses. The viruses are excreted in the droppings and the saliva and can readily infect in-contact birds. In addition, a proportion of the eggs are also infected to pass the virus through to the chick. Chickens receiving their infection through the eggs become tolerant to the virus and do not produce antibodies, whereas those infected after hatching respond with the production of viral antibodies. Chickens tolerant to the virus are more likely to succumb to disease, and if they do not they shed the virus in the eggs more consistently than chickens with a circulating antibody. Lymphoid leucosis is the main form of disease developing after infection with the leucosis virus. It is stated, however, that only about 2 per cent of chickens die from lymphoid leucosis.

Control. There is no treatment and because the infection is transmitted through the egg, management and hygiene methods are unable to control the disease. However, because the viruses are not highly contagious it is relatively easy to prevent infection of a flock from outside. If it is possible to free flocks from infection it is possible to maintain them and their progeny free of infection.

Genetic selection of stock resistant to infection with leucosis viruses creates a population resistant to infection with these viruses, and also reduces the number of birds capable of supporting infection.

Fowl pox

Fowl pox is a virus infection of the pox group that causes lesions in the head and mouth of the bird. It is also possible to find lesions on the legs and mucous membranes such as the cloaca. The lesions on the head and comb are usually wart-like in nature. Those that occur in the mouth are diphtheritic and have the appearance of a cheesy membrane. The general symptoms depend on the area of the body affected. The birds will appear dull and when the mouth is affected may have difficulty in breathing and eating.

When the virus attacks the mucous membranes of the nasal and buccal cavities, mortality can reach as high as 40–50 per cent. The virus causes a marked increase in the output of mucous and this is sometimes referred to as 'wet pox'. The less serious skin form of the disease does not lead to high mortality but can cause a reduced egg production in laying birds.

Diagnosis and treatment. The symptoms are usually certain enough to make a diagnosis of the disease, although if there are doubts a veterinary laboratory can confirm. It is not easy to treat affected birds but it is possible to remove the diphtheritic membranes from the mouth and the area around and then treat with antiseptics and emollients. To prevent the disease it is best to use a live pox vaccine, administered either by wing, web or feather follicle application. Fowl pox is a relatively uncommon condition in temperate climates under intensive conditions but remains as a common complaint in warm climates where the systems are less intensive and may not be scrupulously hygienic.

Egg drop syndrome 1976 (EDS '76)

Since the 1970s it has been known that a variety of viruses, so-called adenoviruses, can infect chickens. While they may have an effect at any time of life, the most serious strains cause sudden and prolonged falls in egg production and a profound effect on egg and shell quality. One particular strain first caused problems in 1976 in broiler breeder parents and has since been designated EDS '76. The condition has also spread to other adult birds but it is in breeders that the effect has been most serious. The syndrome has apparently shown itself in a number of forms. There may be a failure of production to peak as it should or there may be gradual or sudden drops in egg production. The egg production of an affected flock may or may not return to normal. There is also a tendency for lowered hatchability, poor eggshell quality and loss of colour to occur. Diagnosis of this condition requires expert examination since the symptoms can be readily confused with, for example, those of infectious bronchitis and Newcastle disease and perhaps other adenoviruses and infectious avian encephalomyelitis. A vaccine has been produced which has been found completely successful in giving satisfactory protection, e.g. Nobi-vac EDS '76 (Intervet Laboratories Ltd).

Pullet disease ('blue-comb'; 'monocytosis')

Pullet disease was once a very common condition of birds, affecting them soon after they had come into egg production. It has all the signs of a viral infection but has not been definitely established to be so. The symptoms that are visible are usually a marked fall in egg production together with inappetence and lethargy. Some birds may be found dead, dying too quickly to show symptoms, but in most, and especially later cases in the course of the disease, death is preceded by a short period of illness during which purple-coloured combs and wattles are the most noticeable feature, together with diarrhoea and an extremely dejected appearance.

Post-mortem signs are especially associated with abnormalities in the kidneys, which are usually grossly enlarged with crystalline urate deposits. There are also degenerative changes of the birds' ovaries and a general congestion of the carcass including a patchy discolouration of the pectoral muscles. The only useful treatment is to administer tetracylines in the drinking water, ensuring that this is freely available to all the birds. Restriction of food intake may be beneficial for a time and a 'traditional' remedy is to mix in with the diet 10–20 per cent of molasses and to feed the whole diet wet.

Roundheart disease

This is a rather strange condition that occurs in layers on deep litter or straw between the ages of 6 and 12 months. Death is sudden and post mortems show an enlarged (rounded) and discoloured heart. It is believed to be due to a toxic factor but so far none has been discovered and there is no treatment or prevention. Fortunately, it is now uncommon.

Avian tuberculosis

Avian tuberculosis is a disease caused by the bacterium *Mycobacterium tuberculosis avium*. It is a contagious disease passed from bird to bird apparently by contact via the droppings of infected birds.

The disease normally affects older birds when there is a progressive loss of weight (going 'light' as it used to be termed). The birds become unthrifty and the muscles of the breast are reduced in size, exposing the sternum or breast bone. Appetite usually remains normal until the terminal stage of the disease. There may be some lameness and swelling of the joints. The comb and wattles appear pale in colour.

Post-mortem examination reveals lesions which appear as yellowish-white caseous nodules in the liver, spleen and intestines. Laboratory examination can confirm the presence of the disease. No treatment is effective and the disease is best dealt with by good culling of the affected birds combined with a complete depopulation of the house and subsequent disinfection. It is a disease we are likely to see much more of with the emergence of free-range systems, as ground is allowed to become contaminated.

Fowl cholera (avian pasteurellosis)

Fowl cholera is caused by a bacterium *Pasteurella multicoida* and can be a very serious cause of disease in many parts of the world. Infection occurs by the respiratory or alimentary route, which contaminates water, soil and feed. There is an incubation period of 4–10 days and the severity of the condition depends very much on the 'stress' of the birds by poor ventilation, overcrowding and so on. Symptoms in the most acute cases include sudden death in large numbers with signs of cyanosis (purple or mauve colouring) and swelling of the comb and wattles. In the less acute stages there is swelling of the joints and legs causing lameness. Affected birds do not eat or drink and have difficulty in breathing. A thick nasal discharge will be seen, together with a greenish-yellowish diarrhoea. Mortality can be very high indeed, even up to 90 per cent. Diagnosis is made on the basis of the symptoms and on isolation of their organisms. Treatment may be instituted by using antibiotics and other medicines while prevention can be effected by vaccination.

Ascites, oedema or 'water-belly'

Ascites in broilers is an increasingly common condition. The symptoms are a blue comb, feathers ruffled and a grossly enlarged abdomen with fluid. If the bird is opened after death, large quantities of brown-yellow liquid emerge.

Accumulations of fluid, or ascites, occur because the circulation of the blood system may in some way be impaired. This is believed to be primarily due to the very fast growth of broilers, together with insufficient ventilation and too high a stocking rate. Ascites is also associated with *E. coli* septicaemia, probably due to reduced cardiac efficiency. Sometimes losses can be very high and consideration should be given to the following measures to prevent losses.

- Reduce stocking density and increase ventilation.
- Feed a ration of reduced energy and protein to slow the growth rate slightly.
- When an attack occurs treat as for *E. coli* septicaemia, with the same medicine.
- Pay special attention to air circulation to ensure that *fresh incoming* air effectively reaches all the birds and removes stale air promptly.

Avian rhino-tracheitis (turkey rhino-tracheitis; TRT or ART)

A relatively recent disease of turkeys was first described in South Africa but was soon found to be present virtually world-wide. In this disease, the birds develop sudden and serious respiratory symptoms with discharges from the eyes and nose and distension of the sinuses. The most common age of infection is between about 8 and 16 weeks and usually almost all the flock is affected. While it is possible for flocks to recover quickly, secondary infections such as *E. coli* and pasteurella may cause great havoc and losses can easily reach 50 per cent. In laying turkeys there is a severe loss in egg production, which only recovers slowly.

The principal cause of TRT or ART is a pneumovirus which is immuno-suppressive and highly contagious. Unfortunately, the disease is also able to infect chickens, both adult flocks and broilers. In adults it causes a severe loss of egg production and in broilers 'swollen heads' with possibly severe secondary effects. Vaccines are now available and are able to give satisfactory protection. When attacks occur, improved environmental conditions will assist, together with treatment for the secondaries in the usual way.

Duck virus enteritis (DVE)

DVE or duck plague is a further virus infection that is very contagious and affects ducklings between 2 and 6 weeks of age. Symptoms are straightforward – heavy losses up to 100 per cent sometimes, diarrhoea, great thirst and haemorrhage throughout the organs of the body. Protection is by live strains of the vaccine.

Duck virus hepatitis (DVH)

This is an acute, highly contagious disease of young ducklings aged from 2 days to about 4 weeks. The effect is very sudden and the duckling usually dies within an hour or so of the onset of the symptoms, if they are seen at all.

Losses can easily be as much as 90 per cent of a flock, especially if the birds are young. Post-mortem signs are in the liver, which is enlarged and haemorrhagic. The only useful protection from DVH is a vaccine. The most satisfactory procedure is to vaccinate the parent stock, who will pass on protection to the progeny, which should be sufficient.

Intestinal parasites

There are four main intestinal parasites of the chicken as follows.

The tape worm (Davainea proglottina)

Affected birds lose weight and are listless; breathing is rapid and feathers are ruffled and dry. In laying birds there is reduced egg production. At post mortem the intestinal mucosa may be thickened and haemorrhagic and the tape worms are seen. For development of the life cycle the intermediate hosts, such as snails and earthworms, have to be present. Specific treatment should be used where the worms are found. It is understandably only likely that infection will take place under extensive or semi-intensive conditions.

The large round worm (Ascaridia gallic)

This is a large worm up to 80 mm in length, which causes loss of condition, reduced egg production in layers and can even cause death if infection is heavy. Retarded growth, listlessness and diarrhoea are the clearest symptoms. At post mortem the large round worms can be seen in the middle part of the small intestine. The disease is uncommon under hygienic conditions but certainly occurs if the litter is wet and birds are overcrowded.

The hair worm (Capillaria)

The hair worm is a small parasite which affects the upper part of the alimentary tract causing diarrhoea, weakness, reduced egg production and anaemia. Affected birds are listless, weak and lose weight. Hygienic measures and treatment will be as with the other worms.

The caecal worm (Heterakis gallinae)

This is a worm of about 10 mm size which develops in the caeca, affecting chickens and turkeys. Perhaps its most important 'function' is as a transmitter of the parasite causing blackhead (histomoniasis).

Treatments

There are adequate specific treatments to control the round and tape worms, see Table 11.3 for more information on the products.

External parasites

Poultry can be infested with a variety of external parasites such as lice, fleas, and various forms of mites, such as red mite, the depluming mite and scaly leg mite. These mites all burrow into various parts of the birds' skin and create considerable damage. The presence of all these conditions is rather uncommon under modern intensive management, and if general standards of hygiene are high it is doubtful if they will be seen at all. External parasites are more commonly associated with older birds and old-fashioned systems of continuous production. If they do occur, then it is advisable to deal with them energetically as they will have a highly debilitating effect on the birds and may also be associated with the spread of other diseases.

Treatment will depend on the administration of an assortment of effective products, which are listed in Chapter 8. It need hardly be emphasised that if birds are badly infested, especially with mites, they should be culled as they are unlikely to respond very effectively to treatment and they will remain as serious sources of infection.

Common poultry diseases and their treatment

The poultry industries of the world are served by an impressive array of companies producing advanced pharmaceuticals, hygiene products and biologicals. It is no exaggeration to say that without the development of these products modern poultry production as we know it could not exist. However, it is a vital corollary of this fact that the poultry farmer knows generally what is available and makes use of the correct product without delay. Successful enterprises are those which react quickly to any risk or appearance of disease, to prevent or treat. Products can be remarkably cost-effective when they are used in the right circumstances at the correct time. The wise poultry farmer will always consult his professional adviser when he has doubts on the diagnosis or treatment of a disease, or the preventive measures necessary to ensure good health. Table 11.3 lists the most common poultry diseases and gives information on the measures available for their prevention and treatment.

Examples are given of the available commercial products but the absence of some does not imply they are not just as good, merely that it was impossible to include everything world-wide. Most countries have a reasonably reliable system for testing and licensing vaccines and medicines and it is advisable that only officially approved and tested products are used. There are many 'combined' vaccines for poultry incorporating two or three different vaccines and wherever these can be used they are preferable to using vaccines separately. Combined vaccines reduce stress and improve and accelerate the development of immunity.

Table 11.3 A chart of poultry diseases, their prevention and treatment

Parasites and disease	Prevention	Treatment
Adenoviruses (including egg drop syndrome (EDS '76), inclusion body hepatitis (IBH) and turkey haemorrhagicenteritis (THE))	Vaccine will protect against one type, EDS '76 (egg drop syndrome 1976), i.e. Nobi-Vac EDS '76 vaccine (Intervet Laboratories). Vaccines also available from Merial	Non-specific measures such as vitamins, mineral and electrolyte mixtures and often broad-spectrum antibiotics will help in the bird's recovery
Ascites in broilers	Reduce stocking density. Increase ventilation. Improve litter provision. Lower diet intensity to slow growth	Similar to *E. coli*, septicaemia that often occurs at the same time. Potentiated sulphonamides especially useful
Aspergillosis (brooder pneumonia)	Avoid all damp litter and nest material. Check hygiene in all areas of the hatchery	Treat the whole environment with a disinfectant known to be active against fungi, etc., e.g. Farm Fluid S (Antec International) 1:400 or Microsol (Micro-Biologicals 1:100)
Avian clostridial diseases including necrotic enteritis, botulism and gangrenous dermatitis	Hygienic measures within and around buildings need to be improved, together with an improved disinfection and fumigation programme Disinfectants and fumigants should be used with their activity specified against clostridia bacterial spores that are resistant to destruction	Soluble penicillin or semi-synthetic penicillin in drinking water at 0.5 per g per 5 litres of water
Avian influenza (fowl plague)	Blood testing or virus isolation to be followed, usually by slaughter of positive flocks, but can be used as an alternative	No useful treatment, other than supportive antibiotic and vitamin administration

(continued)

Table 11.3 A chart of poultry diseases, their prevention and treatment (*continued*)

Parasites and disease	Prevention	Treatment
Avian leucosis	Blood testing and elimination of infected stock with selection of genetically resistant strains. Also improve all measures of hygiene and isolation	None
Avian mycoplasmosis (chronic respiratory disease – CRD)	Normally eliminated from breeding flocks by blood testing and removal of reactors, also by medication, e.g. with Linco-Spectin 100 (Upjohn). One pack incorporating 100 g of antibiotics per 200 litres of drinking water; or Tylan Soluble (Elanco Products), 2.5 g per 4.5 litres. Vaccination sometimes used but only partially successful	Similar to preventive treatment. In addition, may use tetracycline, macrolides, amino-glycosides and quinolones
Avian pasteurellosis (fowl cholera)	Vaccination by injection, e.g. Pabac Pasteurella vaccine (Fort Dodge) and Pasteurella and Erysipelas vaccine (Hoechst)	Chlorrtetracycline, oxytetracycline, amoxycillin
Avian tuberculosis	Test for reactors and cull infected birds. Ensure hygiene is improved as organism that causes disease is persistent	Nor advocated
Coccidiosis	Medication of ration with a variety of cocciostats, e.g. Elancoban (Elanco Products) 100 g per tonne of feed or 500 g of 20% Premix, broilers only. Also vaccine, e.g. Paracox (Schering-Plough)	Amprol-Plus (Merial) contains amprolium + ethopabate 400 ml in 100 litres of water for 5–7 days, then 100 ml per 100 litres for 14 days

(*continued*)

Table 11.3 A chart of poultry diseases, their prevention and treatment (*continued*)

Parasites and disease	Prevention	Treatment
Duck virus hepatitis	Strict isolation in first few weeks of life and vaccination of parent stock to provide parental immunity, e.g. Hepatovax Live (Merial)	Serum therapy possible and occasionally used
Duck plague (duck virus enteritis)	Cleanliness and hygiene plus vaccination, e.g. use Duck Plague Vaccine Nobilis, or Vaxiduck (Merial)	None
E. coli infections	*E. coli* is usually a secondary infection, thus main efforts must concentrate on prevention of primary disease with vaccination, therapy or good husbandry. Useful medications are potentiated sulphonamides or a variety of water-soluble preparations, such as chlortetracycline (see treatment). *E. coli* vaccines given to breeders to protect their chicks are also used, e.g. Avicolivac (Merial)	Chlortetracycline hydrochloride 0.5 g per 5 litres in drinking water as Aureomycin soluble (Cyanamid) or neomycin as Neobiotic Soluble Powder (Upjohn) up to 0.5 g per 5 litres
Fatty liver and kidney syndrome	Ensure protein and carbohydrate ratio is correct and also that there is sufficient provision in feed of biotin and other vitamin B elements	Administer water-soluble vitamin preparations suitably fortified with biotin
Fowl pox	Vaccination effectively prevents, e.g. Poxine and Poxinet	Administer non-specific broad spectrum antibiotics for secondary infections

(*continued*)

Table 11.3 A chart of poultry diseases, their prevention and treatment (*continued*)

Parasites and disease	Prevention	Treatment
Fowl typhoid and pullorum disease (salmonella galinarium and salmonella pullorum)	Blood testing and culling reactors on a regular basis, combined with improved hygiene and husbandry. Vaccination can be used for typhoid	Potentiated sulphonamides or broad spectrum antibiotics can be used, also Enrofloxacin
Gangrenous dermatitis	Usually associated with broilers after Gumboro disease challenge, so vaccination against this assists. Do not use 'old' litter or over-stock and ensure efficient disinfection between crops	Soluble antibiotics with a broad spectrum of activity, such as amoxycillin
Gumboro disease (infectious bursal disease)	Protect immature birds with live vaccines. To give parental immunity to chicks, give inactivated vaccine to parents	Treat for secondary infections with antibiotics or antibiotic/vitamin mixtures
Histomoniasis (blackhead)	Emtryl Premix (Merial), Sulfuride (Fort Dodge)	Soluble forms of Emtryl
Inclusion body hepatitis	Gumboro vaccination may assist in prevention as Gumboro disease appears to predispose to infection of IBH	Non-specific measures including broad-spectrum antibiotics and vitamins, especially fat-soluble vitamins
Infectious avian encephalomyelitis (epidemic tremor) (*continued*)	A variety of live vaccines given in drinking water at an age of about 15 weeks	No specific treatment, but encourage appetite and drinking by adding vitamin electrolyte mixtures to water

Table 11.3 A chart of poultry diseases, their prevention and treatment (*continued*)

Parasites and disease	Prevention	Treatment
Infectious bronchitis	Vaccination of immature birds by use of live vaccines, e.g. H-120 and H-52 as a coarse spray or in drinking water. Adults may be vaccinated by injection with inactivated vaccines	To curb secondary infections use chlortetracyclines or potentiated sulphonamides. Examples of treatments for secondaries are oxytetracycline or chlortetracycline
Infectious coryza (roup)	Improve environment and hygiene and use vaccine	Haemophilus-sensitive, broad-spectrum antibiotics with supportive administration of soluble vitamins and electrolytes
Infectious laryngotracheitis	Vaccination by injection	Non-specific broad-spectrum antibiotics and soluble vitamins and electrolytes
Infectious stunting syndrome (ISS) (malabsorption syndrome)	No specific vaccines available but some benefit may result from the use of Reo- and Adeno-viruses combined with improved cleaning, hygiene and disinfection	Administer generous quantities of soluble vitamins and electrolytes to assist absorption of essential nutrients
Insect infestation	A wide range of materials exist for dealing with flies, lice, beetles and crawling insects, which are especially liable to infest poultry houses due to their warmth and their cavity construction	

(*continued*)

Table 11.3 A chart of poultry diseases, their prevention and treatment (*continued*)

Parasites and disease	Prevention	Treatment
Marek's disease	Vital to keep chicks away from infection for first few weeks of life. Vaccinate chicks at day-old and again at 10–21 days by intra-muscular route. Vaccine choice dependent on local challenge	No specific treatment, but vitamin and mineral preparations added to drinking water will assist birds
Mites	Disinfection of buildings and equipment with agents with established activity against mites. Removal of wood and other parts where mites are harboured	Use only acaricides that are approved for direct contact with birds by spray, dust or dips
Mycotoxicosis	As source is almost invariably contaminated feedstuffs, contents should be monitored and where risk exists, add a chemical deterrent to feed, e.g. Bio-Add (BP Chemicals)	Little benefit from any medicine, but soluble vitamins and minerals will assist recovery
Necrotic enteritis	Improved hygiene, including phenolic disinfectants and penicillin in feed at a level of 40 g per tonne	Soluble penicillin in water at 0.5 g per 5 litres of water, or broad-spectrum antibiotics
Newcastle disease (fowl pest)	Variety of vaccines protect, e.g. Hitchner B_1, and Ma 5 by spray droplet or water medication, largely for young or growing stock, and inactivated oil-adjuvant vaccines by injection. Primarily for layers or breeders	No treatment effective against the virus of Newcastle disease, but treatment for secondaries under *E. coli* infections

(*continued*)

Table 11.3 A chart of poultry diseases, their prevention and treatment (*continued*)

Parasites and disease	Prevention	Treatment
Perosis	Ensure a balanced ration, sufficient especially in manganese, other minerals and phosphorus	As prevention, administer extra soluble vitamins and minerals to assist utilisation of feed
Roundworms	Normal hygienic measures during and between batches of chickens on litter	Piperazine hydrochloride. Mebendazole: Benenvet 5% (Janssen)
Salmonellosis	General prevention relies on good hygiene and security of poultry sites, ensuring hygienic feedstuffs, and serology on flocks, with elimination or treatment of those infected. After a site is infected, it is essential to destroy all possible vectors of disease, i.e. rats, mice, litter beetles and insects. Vaccine against *S. enterididis*	Enrofloxacin and sensitive broad-spectrum antibiotics
Turkey rhino-tracheitis (TRT) of turkeys and swollen head syndrome of chicken	Vaccination given from day-old onwards when flock is at risk	Generally concentrates on secondary infection, e.g. furazolidone or potentiated sulphonamides, or broad-spectrum antibiotics in feed or in drinking water
Viral arthritis (tenosynovitis)	Live and inactivated vaccines available for good protection	Benefits are derived from the use of broad-spectrum antibiotics, soluble vitamins and electrolytes

12 Turkeys

Turkeys are no longer eaten on special occasions; they are now a true round-the-year attraction and very good value indeed. There is quite a range of turkeys produced for the market. The smallest 'mini' turkey finished at about 12 weeks, weighs 4.5 kg (10 lb) or the medium weight ('midi') at 16 weeks weighs 6.5 kg (14.5 lb). Then for the more traditional festive or, more likely, catering trade the heavier bird is required, which will be kept from 18–30 weeks and will weigh from 9 kg (18 lb) to 15 kg (35 lb). In addition, the industry is marketing turkey portions, turkey rolls and turkey sausages and other 'so-called' added-value products incorporating turkey meat, thus supplying the consumer with a very wide range of turkey products. The world production of turkeys continues to rise consistently year by year. The smaller birds are kept very much like broilers in similar housing, although usually not with such a fully controlled environment, whereas the heavier birds can be kept quite satisfactorily in simple housing of the pole-barn type or even outdoors.

Unlike the domestic fowl, which almost invariably breeds naturally, modern strains of turkey are so cumbersome and broad-breasted that natural mating is at least difficult and often impossible. Use is therefore made of artificial insemination, the males being 'milked' for semen to inseminate hens approximately once every 2 weeks, but often more frequently and even weekly. Most of the modern hybrids are based on two foundation breeds, the Broad-breasted Bronze and the Beltsville White.

Rearing systems

Turkeys are brooded and weaned off heat at 8–10 weeks of age under intensive conditions, following which they may continue the growing period of 24 weeks or more in confinement, or they can be moved to good clean pastures to encourage their natural grazing habits. Short-term rearing from day-old to 16 weeks is almost always undertaken in controlled-environment houses. Breeding stock may be reared extensively or semi-intensively but although the capital cost of an enterprise of this sort is cheap, running costs are high and may be uneconomic.

Separate quarters are recommended for different age groups and the 'all-in, all-out' system whereby one age group is reared to killing age and the premises depopulated and cleaned is strongly advocated for turkeys, as for domestic fowls.

The principal brooding system involves the use of either solid or wire floors. Floor brooding on a litter of wood shavings or other material requires a large floor area, which must be free from draughts and the litter must be maintained in a dry condition to minimise the risk of parasitic infestations. Well-insulated and ventilated houses are required with supplementary heating to maintain a house temperature of 25°C (77°F) during the early stages of brooding.

Tier brooding cages are an alternative and once popular system, being especially made to give adequate headroom and unobstructed access to food and water troughs, taking 50–70 poults to 3 weeks of age. They involve higher capital outlay than is needed for floor brooding, but allow greater concentration per unit of floor space. They are easily serviced and may be installed in many conversions. Less costly are frames of weldmesh fitted in a small unit or compartment of a house.

It is well to emphasise that early mortality in turkey poults due to lack of drinking or feeding is a constant problem that has to be prevented by good management and by providing the best equipment giving readily accessible food and water and plenty of bright lighting.

For the weaning stage cooler battery cages may be used in a room temperature of 16°C (60°F) declining to 10°C (50°F). Alternatively an outdoor static hay box with a stronger wire floor above a droppings pit will take 35–40 poults to 8 weeks old. Wire floor verandahs added to wire floor houses provide a further increase in floor space. The use of wire floors dispenses with litter problems, separates the poults from their droppings and permits free circulation of air around the poults, but the complexity of the wire floor systems, together with high labour requirements, makes them increasingly unattractive, except in limited circumstances.

Turkeys react to changes of environment and care is needed when these are made, especially when the change is extreme – such as a move from a wire or slatted floor to litter. In general, simple and standardised rearing on the floor is replacing other techniques and disease control is achieved by vaccine and medicines.

Growing and fattening range systems

Some flocks are still reared on range and indeed the range system is clearly increasing as modern fashions dictate. Clean land which has not carried poultry or turkeys for 2 years is essential and is best divided into paddocks of not more than 500 turkeys with ring fencing some 3 m high as protection from predators. Turkeys are extremely hardy when the feathers are 'bloomed' and on range they need only simple housing or shelters. Open or covered roosts and straw bale shelters will suffice. Some flocks may find security in a wire compound or farm building. Feeding and drinking equipment needs protection from weather, farm animals, wild birds and predators. Although more expensive to operate, the fold units of 20–40 turkeys provide better control with more even grazing and manuring of the lands.

Intensive systems

These must provide adequate fresh air and floor space for growing stock. These requirements are met at low cost in the 3 m high wire netting or straw bale turkey compound, with open-air perches. Food and water troughs are placed outside and the compound area is covered with straw or wood shavings, but in a wet season this system is costly to operate. The turkey yard has the same basic arrangement but the perches are under a lean-to or old farm building. The pole shed is a completely covered compound constructed of rough poles, railway sleepers or timber posts carrying a roof of wire netting overlaid with building felt or corrugated roofing material. Ends and back walls are fully or partially protected with straw bales, polythene or other sheeting but the remainder is covered with large mesh netting. Water troughs and supplementary food troughs are accessible from the front. No perches are provided and a 13 m × 13 m section usually accommodates 300–500 turkeys.

Verandah and wire cage systems are both used for off-the-ground rearing in small units on limited land. Many of the modern units used for large-scale rearing of part grown turkeys have efficient insulation, mechanical ventilation, supplementary heating and lighting to provide a controlled environment in all seasons and it is this arrangement, similar to that used with the chicken, which is gradually replacing all other arrangements.

Bearing in mind the rapid growth of turkeys, the minimum space requirements shown in Table 12.1 should not be economised on any further and more space is *always* advantageous.

Poults grow rapidly and in consequence need increased headroom under the brooders, floor space, feeding space and ventilation in the house. It should be recognised that poults at 4 weeks are 12 times their day-old weight and at 8 weeks are three times their 4-week weight.

After the young turkeys are hardened at 6–8 weeks and probably moved to new growing quarters the aim should be to maintain unchecked growth.

Table 12.1 Space requirements (per bird)

Brooders	Hover units		0.008 m^2
	Suspended heaters		0.013 m^2
	Battery brooders		0.016 m^2
Intensive housing	Floor space	0–4 weeks	0.08 m^2
		5–8 weeks	0.12 m^2
		9–14 weeks	0.24 m^2
		15 weeks to killing	0.30–0.48 m^2
Pole sheds		15 weeks to killing (hens)	0.24 m^2
		(stags)	0.40 m^2
Compounds			0.48–0.72 m^2
Range	Clean pasture		450 turkeys per hectare
Feeding trough space	Minimum per 100 turkeys		
2 weeks	4 m		
3–4 weeks	6 m	with tubular feeders use	
5–6 weeks	7 m	2–3 per 100 birds each	
7–16 weeks	9 m	holding 13.62 kg of feed	
17 weeks to killing	12 m		
Drinkers	Minimum per 100 turkeys		
0–4 weeks	3 × 2 founts		
4–8 weeks	2 m		
8–24 weeks	3 m		

At this time turkeys go through a stage known as 'shooting the red' when the head parts become a bright colour as the bird matures, and if the hens and stags have not already been separated, this is a good time to do it.

Turkeys to be reared in confinement should have their beaks trimmed to prevent vice, just prior to moving, but it is best not to make any changes in management until the birds are settled. They are most satisfactorily kept in small groups of up to 250 birds, with adequate floor and feeding space for their rapid growth in the next 3–4 months. Where perches are not used, a few bales of straw will help prevent the young turkeys from herding and smothering when kept in large groups. In close confinement a high standard of stockmanship is demanded since vices are more prevalent and disease risks are increased. Cleanliness at feeding and drinking sites and a liberal supply of clean litter is essential. Poor results are often due to overcrowding and inadequate ventilation, which seem to be common errors in management in spite of all the recent evidence of their harmful effects.

Breeding turkeys

Breeders are maintained in two ways. One system is to maintain them on the floor in one of the several ways mentioned earlier. It will be appreciated that controlled-environment housing is gaining in acceptance because with its control of all conditions, including lighting, as with breeding chickens, it has enabled much greater efficiency and productivity. Hens and stags may be kept together for natural mating or hens and stags may be kept separately and insemination carried out artificially. An alternative arrangement is to house the hens and stags as individuals in cages kept in a house with a well-controlled environment. Such a system gives maximum control of the birds and easier handling and is a system that continues to gain in popularity. The following minimum areas should be provided, but there is much to be said for increasing the space given to the birds if at all possible.

Hens and stags maintained on the floor in groups for natural mating	20 kg/m^2
Stags on the floor for artificial breeding	$1 \text{ m}^2/\text{bird}$
Hens in cages	30 kg/m^2
Stags in cages	1 m^2 per bird
Birds out of doors	20 m^2 per bird

Feeding

Management of turkeys is similar to that of the domestic fowl with regard to housing, environment, lighting, hygiene and disease control but feeding is so important that the differences should be carefully noted (see Chapters 3 and 4). The slowness in getting young poults to accept their food is well known and they must be coaxed to eat by making sure they can easily see the food and by having plenty of feeding points.

The same applies to water. Bright lighting is essential. All growing systems supply food *ad lib* except where there is added grain, which is given at special times in measured amounts. With outdoor methods no more food should be given than can be cleared up fairly soon after feeding as otherwise wild birds or vermin consume it. Turkey poults are supplied with food containing at least 24 per cent of crude protein for the first 8 weeks of life, reducing this level to 20 per cent at 12 weeks and 16 per cent at 16 weeks. A finishing ration for the heavier bird will have a protein percentage of about 13 per cent.

Substances similar to those in chicken rations are used. A poult 'starter' ration is fed up to 8 weeks and a 'grower' ration, which may be supplemented with grain if desired, is fed thereafter. The finishing ration is usually introduced about 3 weeks before the birds are to be marketed. Emphasis must be placed on the importance of insoluble grit for turkeys, as for chickens, especially when fed a grain diet.

The maintenance of health

The first stage of vulnerability for the turkey is at the very beginning of its life. They are much more inclined to perish than chicks or ducklings, for no apparent reason, although it may be emphasised that they have very good sight. Thus, they need to be surrounded by water and food, plenty of light and adequate warmth, at least 35°C (95°F) at a house heat of about 25°C (77°F). It is desirable that this temperature difference of 10°C between the brooder area and the house is maintained. The intensification of turkey production has led to a considerable increase in the disease incidence. The chapters on the prevention and treatment of disease give adequate coverage of the diseases and should be studied carefully if health is to be taken seriously. What must be stressed here is that prevention is, as always, the best approach and can start very soon after hatching by administering vaccines, including rhino-tracheitis, pox, pasteurellosis and erysipelas. Whether some or all of these are necessary will depend on the local incidence. If rearing is to be done in an area where there are many turkeys, full vaccinal protection may be required, but in an isolated location little or none may be necessary. This illustrates only too well the importance of choosing the right area to keep turkeys, although sadly, poultry producers, for logistical reasons, can rarely be persuaded away from their suicidal tendency to bunch together, not unlike the birds they keep!

At present probably the worst disease affecting turkeys is rhino-tracheitis and is the latest viral infection to become a scourge for turkeys throughout most of the world. It has a really devastating effect on flocks of any age and after the initial viral damage, all the usual secondary viruses and bacteria can wreak great havoc. Losses of up to 30 per cent can easily occur, accompanied by massive losses of productivity in those birds that stay alive. Treatment with medicine to reduce losses will usually help but sometimes hardly at all. Thus, if there is a likelihood of birds being challenged a full programme of protection by vaccination is essential. Some help, or even a great deal, may result from improving the environment by providing more space, better air movement and ventilation, and a fresh covering of good quality litter. It should hardly be necessary to emphasise this again but I do not apologise for stating my belief that if we had no vaccines or medicines we could perhaps be even more successful in rearing turkeys, as with all livestock, by relying on good feeding, housing hygiene, husbandry and management.

13 Ducks

The market for table ducks is steadily increasing. Egg layers, however, remain in decline as the strong flavour of the duck egg remains unattractive to the consumer. On the other hand, the table duck is being managed under increasingly sophisticated conditions that improve the value of the product for the housewife. Table ducks can make extremely fast growth, a live weight of 3–3.5 kg (6.5–7.5 lb) being attainable in 7–8 weeks at a food conversion efficiency of about 2:1.

Breeds

The Aylesbury was by tradition the supreme table breed; it is a white feathered light-boned duck with creamy white flesh, the adult drakes weighing about 4.5 kg (10 lb) and the females about 4.1 kg (9 lb). However, its popularity has been challenged by the Pekin, as a result of genetic improvement of this breed in the USA. The Pekin is a smaller bird (about 0.45 kg (1 lb) lighter at the adult stage, but it is more fertile, a better layer and a more economical grower.

Two other table breeds are the Pennine, which has a good carcase quality and better egg production than the Aylesbury, and the White table duck, which is claimed to have a high percentage of meat. The two common egg-laying varieties, the Khaki Campbell and Indian Runner, are both prolific producers, an egg a day for a year being quite attainable. Modern hybrid strains of both egg and table birds are being developed from existing breeds. They have the same advantage as the chicken hybrids in that they combine the best features of two or more breeds, yet still produce a high degree of vigour and uniformity.

Breeding

The duck appears to respond to the lighting stimulus in the same way as the chicken; that is, breeding activity is induced by an incremental increase in the period of light in each 24-hour period. Breeding pens should contain one male for every eight females: they should be made up in groups at least a month before eggs are required for hatching. Great care should be taken when designing accommodation to ensure that nest boxes can be kept clean, especially in view of the traditional hazard of duck breeding – infection with the salmonella group of bacteria. The nesting material must be changed frequently and the eggs collected soon after laying, then washed in a combined detergent and antiseptic solution at a temperature slightly above that of the eggs. Thereafter the eggs should be dried, fumigated and stored at 14–15°C (58–60°F) and a relative humidity of 80 per cent.

Usually eggs are not used for hatching until the ducks have been laying for about 6–8 weeks. Incubation requires a temperature of 37.5°C (99.5°F) and a humidity of 75 per cent 31°C or 87°F wet bulb.

Feeding

Table 13.1 gives examples of three suitable rations for ducks through their life cycle. It is considered a preferable technique to feed all three rations in pelleted form.

In the USA growing stock are often fed rations containing higher protein levels (18–20 per cent). It is important to maintain the correct ratio between the energy and crude protein levels and the figure should be 140:1 for the starter feed and 160:1 for the growers.

A substitute feeding regime for the young stock is a starter diet for the first 2 weeks, preferably in the form of crumbs, alternatively as a wet mash. During this time a trough space of 50 mm per duckling should be allowed. From 2 weeks onwards the 'grower' food is best given as a pellet and the trough space increased up to 100 mm per duck. Birds to be kept for breeding are given pelleted feed and often grain as a night feed with a total intake of 0.3–0.4 kg (6–8 oz) per day, which is similar to the food consumed by the adult. In the management of ducks it is most important that the food is given in troughs which are capacious enough to enable the birds to make use of the shovelling action of their beaks. Ducks of all ages drink large quantities of water and while this must be provided, vessels must be designed so they can be kept clean to avoid bacterial infections.

Brooding

Young ducklings can be brooded by floor and battery systems similar to those described for chickens but at slightly lower starting temperatures of 30°C (86°F). Three-tier battery units measuring 1200 mm × 600 mm × 250 mm

Table 13.1 Examples of duck rations (kg per tonne mix)

	Starter ration 0–2 weeks	Grower ration 0–6 weeks	Finisher ration 6 weeks to finishing	Breeder ration	Holding ration*
Wheat meal (coarse)	500	423	600	433	800
Maize meal (fresh)	267	329	300	300	–
Barley meal (fine)	–	100	–	–	165
Fishmeal	113	50	31	67	–
Soya-bean meal	100	54	–	67	–
Meat and bone meal	8	25	50	33	22
Grass meal	–	–	–	33	–
Limestone (flour or granules	10	10	10	60	–
Dicalcium phosphate	–	7	–	–	–
Fat	–	–	6	–	–
Supplement (vitamin/mineral)	13	13	13	13	13
Calculated analysis					
Crude protein %	20.2	15.5	13.3	17.0	11.3
ME kcal/kg	2885	2877	2965	2694	2825
Ca %	1.24	1.12	0.99	3.1	0.21

*Suitable for breeding ducks between 8–20 weeks of age and for moulting between laying periods.

and holding 25 ducklings to 3 weeks of age are frequently used, but many growers prefer a single-tier arrangement. A unit measuring 1050 mm × 2100 mm will take about 100 ducklings for the first week of life. Ducklings brooded on the floor can be kept in a variety of buildings, the traditional system being a long narrow house which opens on each side of a centre passage. With this arrangement the ducklings can later be released for the fattening period into an outside run on each side of the building. Litter materials include straw, sawdust, shavings, peat moss and sand, but the large quantities of water that ducks drink and therefore void present a severe problem with almost any form of bedding. That is why a wire base, as in tier brooders, follow-on cages and simple wire-floored systems, tends to be used for brooding and subsequent periods. A suitable wire floor for the first 4 weeks consists of a 12.5-mm mesh of 8 gauge.

Rearing and fattening

This is the period from about 4 weeks onwards when ducks would traditionally be put indoors. They are placed in groups of about 200 at a density of 5000 to a hectare and they should be on light sandy soil such as is found in the Brecklands of Norfolk in the UK, where a high proportion of the industry is based. The pens must be moved frequently and require a light fencing only about 1 m high; shelter from the worst effects of the weather can be provided by wind breaks and covers of straw bales and corrugated iron. There are, however, serious doubts on the economics of outdoor systems, especially during the winter and an increasing amount of indoor fattening is carried out both in winter and summer. This is often done on straw bedding and at other times on welded wire or slats, 25 m mesh of 8 gauge being suitable and allowing up to 0.1 m^2 of floor space per bird by the end of the fattening period. In indoor systems the ducks are frequently provided with access to outside yards of asphalt or concrete or merely well-sanded earth. These appear to have considerable benefits in that they give the birds more room at low costs, and they can certainly be advocated provided that the base is well drained and (if permanent floor is not used) measures are taken to rest and disinfect the soil. Wire-floored verandahs can also be incorporated with all indoor housing systems, being a cheap and safe way of providing fresh air and exercise.

Mention should be made of one or two less common arrangements. For the rearing of breeding birds colony housing may be used, the ducks being reared in a small pen at one end of a house and moved into larger pens as they grow. Grass pens in conjunction with slatted floor houses are also used for small groups, either for rearing or breeding. Occasionally hay box brooders, in which the ducklings' warmth is maintained and retained in a nest of hay, rather than by the use of artificial heat, are used for the period from 2–5 weeks.

The space allowances are shown in Table 13.2. They can be taken only as a general guide to the needs of the birds. It is never wrong and indeed virtually always advantageous to give more and this is especially true in small groups. Outside a space allowance of up to 1 m^2 is a reasonable figure.

Table 13.2 Space allowance per duck(ling) – indoors

Age (weeks)	Space allowance (m^2)
1–3	0.045
3–4	0.068
4–5	0.09
5–6	0.113
6–8	0.18

Adults

A variety of arrangements of equal success can be used for housing adult breeding birds. Contrary to common belief there seems no virtue in providing swimming water, but cool *ad lib* drinking water is necessary.

The simplest method of all is to put the laying flocks on free range at a rate of about 750 ducks to the hectare. If the pasture is reasonably good this enables some economies in feed and the ducks can benefit from access to ground, such as marshes which could not support other livestock. While adults can be kept outside without any form of protection this is not advisable economically, particularly in winter, and there is also an increased health risk. Housing can, however, be simple timber or hardboard construction with a floor of well-drained concrete or wire mesh. An allowance of 0.2–0.3 m² per bird is sufficient.

Various other semi-intensive or intensive arrangements may be used. A simple system seen commonly in Europe consists of rows of narrow pens each containing about 8–10 breeding or laying birds, the ground being sloped to one end and usually having a sandy base. A small shelter is provided at one end.

Nowadays, however, the trend is towards the maintenance of adult breeding stock or laying stock in controlled-environment intensive housing similar to that used for chickens. A suitable system is to have the house divided into slatted areas containing the drinkers and a bedded area, usually of straw and shavings. Housing may even be heated in an attempt to reduce the amount of straw used by increasing the drying effect of the air. Ventilation rates in intensive housing must also be maintained at a high rate and automatic fan systems are favoured when stocking rates are high. For intensive housing small flocks of about 200–250 birds are recommended. Nest boxes should be provided at the rate of one nest to every three ducks. They are usually placed on the floor around the walls or against the partitions between pens.

In order to obtain a constant supply of ducklings throughout the year one of two arrangements may be employed. Either the ducks are introduced to produce hatching eggs for as long as possible – up to about 25–30 weeks – or they are allowed to lay for about 3 months, then force-moulted and rested for a similar period, after which there will normally be another laying period. Moulting can be induced in several ways, by moving the birds, by feeding a grain-only diet or by gradually reducing the lighting periods.

In the successful management of ducks, good housing, coupled with high standards of nutrition, are the cornerstones of a profitable programme but hygiene is especially important as a supporting procedure. Traditional systems, in the main, are not satisfactory under the more intensive regimes now favoured and improved standards of health control and environmental regulations are tending to increase indoor management and reduce the popularity of the outdoor arrangements.

Maintaining good health

Unlike chickens or turkeys, few vaccinations are normally required for ducks. Vaccination against duck virus hepatitis (DVH) (see also Chapter 11) may, however, be advisable. DVH vaccine should be used only on farms that have experienced a previous incidence of the disease and the same is true when vaccines are used for duck virus enteritis (DVE) and pasteurellosis.

We rely very heavily on good 'quality control' to keep disease away. Ducks quickly make an area into a mess with a strong likelihood of a build-up of infection occurring. The desirability of giving generous space allowances, good underfoot conditions, a healthy environment and constant attention to hygiene, cannot be exaggerated. If conditions are bad there may be an upsurge in fungal infections which are difficult to treat, and in breeders egg-borne disease can create enormous losses. There is also the possibility of ducks being infected with parasites, especially when they are on pasture. The effect of parasitic infection, as with bacterial infections, may be sub-clinical so that no obvious signs of disease are seen, but nevertheless there will be heavy losses due to poor productivity. If the duck owner has the slightest indication that his birds are so affected, a sample of mortality and/or live 'culls' should be submitted for examination to a veterinary laboratory or it is even better if the veterinarian can visit the premises and examine all relevant aspects.

14 Geese

The production of geese has changed little over many years and there has been little attempt at genetic improvement. The common types in this country are English grey, English white and English grey back. They are based essentially on the original breeds of Embden and Toulouse with an admixture of others. While there are considerable variations, ganders reach weights of 8–9 kg and a goose weighs about 7 kg. Egg production varies between 30 and 80 eggs in a season.

Breeding

Selection for breeding should be made on the usual basis; that is, egg production, fertility, hatchability, viability and conformation. It is important to make up the breeding pen (or 'set') of geese with care as they will not mate and breed satisfactorily unless they are in harmony with each other and have had some weeks living together. It is advisable to make up the sets about 2 months before the season's breeding in the spring. They can stay together for years; there are plenty of records of geese living together and breeding for two decades at least. The mating ratio is best at four or five geese to one gander, although a wider ratio is not infrequently used. Each set should be allocated to a separate house when it is made up and confined within a run separated from other sets. Thereafter, once established, a number of sets can be run together in a paddock.

Incubation

Goose eggs require between 29 and 32 days' incubation. They may be hatched naturally, either under a broody goose or a hen. It is a reasonably simple procedure – the broody 'mother' is put in a separate coop on an earth floor and bedding of straw and fed and watered regularly. The eggs should be turned once a day and the nests have a little warm water run under them to ensure the eggs do not get too dry. If the eggs are incubated artificially, the machine should be run at the same temperature and humidity as chicken eggs and turned not less than once a day. A goose egg will take up the space of about four chicken eggs. Procedures for candling eggs and removing infertiles should be followed in the same way as with incubation generally.

Brooding

If geese are brooded naturally the goose or hen 'mother' will remain with them as long as required.

If reared artificially, similar facilities can be provided as for turkeys, chicken or ducks. A temperature of 38°C (100°F) is the normal starting figure, whether the goslings are kept on wire floors or solid floors with litter. As the droppings from goslings tend to be rather wet it is vital for their good health to ensure that the litter is tended and cleared or topped-up to keep the condition healthy and dry. Artificial heat will not be needed for more than 3 weeks, but the goslings should be let out onto short grass as soon after hatching as possible. While it is advisable to keep the birds in a fairly restricted area for the first week or two, they may soon be given real 'free range'. The only housing required is a basic shelter with a sound, dry floor. It is of benefit if the birds have access to a pond but it is not an essential requirement.

Nutrition

The basic nutritional requirement for the profitable farming of geese is to provide quality grass, short, succulent and nutritious.

It is not a good procedure to put the geese on long fibrous grass as this has little value. At the beginning of their life the goslings may be started on duck crumbs or mini-pellets. This is better than the more traditional mash

Table 14.1 Approximate live-weight for age

Age	Weight (kg)
Day-old	0.10
4 weeks	1.30
8 weeks	2.80
12 weeks	3.70
16 weeks	4.50
20 weeks	4.90
24 weeks	5.50
28 weeks	6.50

Table 14.2 Goose diets (kg/tonne)

	Starter	Grower	Breeder
Wheat (coarse ground)	300	350	250
Barley (fine ground)	200	300	200
Maize (fresh ground)	300	200	300
Dried grass	50	–	–
Meat and bone meal	20	30	60
Fish meal	50	30	60
Soya-bean meal	60	70	80
Limestone (flour or granules)	10	10	40
Dicalcium phosphate	5	5	5
Salt	5	5	5
Vitamin/mineral supplement	12	12	12
Calculated analysis			
Crude protein	16	15.6	18
Energy, kcal/kg	2765	2788	2733

feeding, although the latter system can be used if preferred. This food may be provided *ad lib* for the first few weeks and should have the addition of some small size insoluble grit. The birds must not be overstocked. A reasonable maximum stocking rate for permanent pasture is about 100 geese to a hectare. However, a more fruitful and intensive way of rearing the geese is to stock them much more heavily, up to 600 birds per hectare, and to keep moving them around at 4-weekly intervals to new ground. Geese for the table will be ready at 10–12 weeks, especially if good quality supplementary feed is provided. After the goslings have reached approximately 8 weeks of age, the mixture may be usefully supplemented with some whole grains. The feeding of the breeders depends on some quite different factors. During the winter months the birds will need to be fed a simple maintenance diet, usually a mixture of wheat, barley, maize and dried grass. It is desirable to give the breeders a diet supplemented with adequate vitamins and minerals. It is not easy to be dogmatic about the quantities of food used but one can keep a careful watch on the condition of the geese. Ensure that all birds have access to the litter. Table 14.2 is a sample of Ministry of Agriculture UK approved and recommended diets for 'home mixers'.

The future

At present there is a limited demand for geese and production has actually been in decline until quite recently, when there has been some sign of revival.

The fall in demand has probably been due to the poor quality of the products, with poor quantity of meat and excessive fat. Nevertheless, the meat has a most attractive 'natural' flavour and if more attention is paid to the correct feeding and breeding the profitability could return and the rearing of geese could form a useful adjunct to a mixed farming operation. As with the production of quail, improved productivity can be achieved by applying our increasing knowledge on poultry production in general. For example, geese are traditionally seasonal layers but investigations have shown that out-of-season production can be stimulated by the use of a 16- or 17-hour day. A period of short days (6–8 hours) needs to be given to breeding geese before the 16-hour day for a good effect.

Geese are relatively free of disease but they should be checked for parasites, especially the gizzard worm, and duly treated if necessary. Management techniques can reduce the chances of such diseases, by reducing the stocking density or moving the geese more frequently. Improving selection by better breeding techniques and hygiene and hatchery practice can also reap considerable dividends. None of these proposals will compromise the unique, special flavour and natural methods that commend the goods for the table.

15 Quail

Quail production throughout the world is sharply on the increase both for meat and egg consumption. While they are still considered to be largely luxury foods, improvements in the genetic quality of the birds has led to better productivity and a more satisfactory economic outlook for their more widespread demand. The future of quail production indeed looks encouraging world-wide. The most commonly used breed, especially in the UK, is the Japanese quail (*Coturnix coturnix Japonica*). The average females weigh about 250 g, the male a little less. Egg weight is some 14 g. Quail lay some 200 eggs a year and the young birds are ready for the table at about 40 days at a live-weight of 250 g.

Housing and environment

Quail can be grown in either cages or on litter. While the traditional practice is to brood in one area and transfer to a grower house at 2–3 weeks, it is really much better to remove the unnecessary stress of a move in a table-quail's very short life. Whichever system is used, the arrangement and techniques are similar to those for chickens and brooders; cages and housing and equipment are adapted. The correct ambient temperature is vital for good quail production and the birds should be brooded at 35–36°C (95–97°F) gradually reducing over 3 weeks to 20°C (68°F). A good start is vital and it is best to commence with feed and water in plastic apple trays, weaning them on to automatic cups or nipple drinkers shortly afterwards.

The birds should be floor-brooded at 150 birds per square metre, reduced at 2 weeks to 100 birds in the same space. If the birds are reared in cages, they can be housed at a rate of double that provided for the chickens. Light intensity is most important and it should be very bright to start with (60–70 lux), reduced to about 10 lux by 3 weeks, where lighting is fully controlled. The birds can be given 23 hours' light a day, as it is best to give them an hour's darkness from day-old, so they will be accustomed to a power or lighting failure and will not panic if plunged into darkness abruptly.

With birds reared on the floor the best litter is soft wood shavings or chopped straw. Special care must be taken to see that the litter has been stored in a dry state since dampness can cause aspergillosis and this respiratory disease can easily cause havoc amongst quail since they are more susceptible than most birds. If it is preferred to rear in cages, ordinary chicken tier brooders may be used at a density of about twice that used for chicks; special tier brooders and follow-on brooders are also made for quail.

Feeding

Quail being reared for meat are usually given *ad lib* turkey rations. Most growers use a turkey super-starter ration from day-old to 14 days and thereafter there is a change to turkey starter to the finish. The best form of feed is a small crumb, especially small in the first stages of the birds' life and smaller than is usual for turkey poults or chicks. By 40 days the birds will be near mature weight and this is the time to kill. They will have a food conversion efficiency of approximately 2.2 from hatching to finishing. The feeding of breeders requires a different regime. The birds require a diet of 20 per cent protein and 11.5 MJ/ME/kg. In practice those types of ration given to a light hybrid chicken breeder will be satisfactory, although some farmers provide a proprietary game breeders ration. The birds will require approximately 25 g per head per day. As there is a limited demand for quail eggs for human consumption, some birds will be kept for this purpose and can be given the same feed as light hybrid chicken layers.

Breeding

Selection of breeders is usually made on the basis of inspection, weight and condition. The main requirement is to have birds in perfect health and showing good uniformity. The birds should be obtained from known recommended lines with good egg laying ability, viability and hatchability. It is most important to avoid inbreeding during the operation of a breeding programme. Using criss-cross breeding, taking males and females from alternate families, inbreeding is avoided and a measure of hybrid vigour is maintained, yet good characteristics are retained. It is wise to keep a minimum of six lines and preferably more to assist with this programme.

When making up the breeding pens the best procedure is to have two or three males with between six and nine females. Such a pen of no more than 12 birds is very satisfactory, but it is currently more common to place the birds in larger units. The females should keep up production for the best part of a year. Fertility will fade quite markedly, however, after 5–6 months but the position can be improved by replacing the males in the breeding pens at about 5 months.

As quail are hot weather birds, in the breeding pen the temperature should be maintained at least at 20°C (68°F). Lighting schedules can be similar to those advised elsewhere for breeders.

Incubation

Quail eggs are extremely delicate and must be handled with great care. Many breeders prefer to dip them in a sanitising solution before storage, which should be 16–20°C (59–68°F) and a relative humidity of no less than 75 per cent. They should not be stored for more than 7 days.

Quail eggs can be incubated in the same machines as for chicken eggs but the equipment will take double the number. Eggs take just under 16 days from setting to pipping and a further 10 hours from pipping to hatching. The regime advised is as follows in the machines. At the start the temperature should be 37.5°C (99.5°F) and the relative humidity 87 per cent (wet bulb temperature 30.6°C (87°F)). At about 15 days the temperature should be reduced to 37°C (98.6°F) and the relative humidity increased to 90 per cent (32.3°C wet bulb temperature). The temperature should be changed to 37.2°C (99°F) at take-off and the relative humidity increased to 90 per cent (27.6°C wet bulb temperature). Eggs must be turned up to seven times a day if it is not an automatic turning machine.

Traditional housing arrangement

For the small and traditional grower the housing designs shown in Figures 15.1 and 15.2 are strongly recommended by an undoubted expert on quail, Mr G.E.S. Robbins (see Further Reading). The quail breeder house, Figure 15.1, is easily constructed from timber and oil-tempered hardboard for outside use. The food and water are replenished without upsetting the birds. In the breeder house small nest boxes are placed so that the access for collection of the eggs is through the small hinged flap shown in the diagram. Also shown are simple quail pens (Figure 15.1) in which the quail can be grown on the floor and a recommended design is shown of a range of quail aviaries (Figure 15.2).

Health and productivity

Quail are affected by a range of diseases which is very similar to other poultry but under most conditions, with good hygiene and management, losses are small as enterprises are generally modest in size. Some of the most common conditions are listed below (for details on treatment consult the earlier chapters on diseases).

Fig. 15.1 Designs for (a) quail breeder house and (b) quail pens.

- Respiratory conditions due to *Aspergillus fumigatus,* mycoplasma and secondary infections – very similar to chronic respiratory disease of chickens, including pasteurella.
- Intestinal disorders due to bacterial build-up, the commonest being clostridia, *E. coli* and staphylococcus.
- Skin disorders such as mites are common under bad hygienic conditions.
- Parasitic conditions may also occur ranging from coccidiosis to blackhead, intestinal and bronchial parasites.

Fig. 15.2 Design of a range of six quail aviaries constructed by Keith Howman.

The future for quail

The market in Europe and especially in France shows that there is a good potential for specialist markets, and if productivity can be improved these interesting prospects will open up in the future. There is no reason why very great advances should not be achieved by applying better breeding techniques, enhanced methods in the hatchery and improved environmental conditions for keeping the breeders and growing the young birds to maturity.

There is also a need to improve hygiene measures in line with those used in other sections of the poultry industry as most of the diseases that occur are avoidable by better management and methods.

16 The Management of Poultry in Hot Climates

Large poultry units are being increasingly developed in areas of high temperature that are not traditional to advanced methods of husbandry and special techniques should be considered for the satisfactory management of birds under these conditions.

Housing and environment

Naturally ventilated (or convection housing)

There is no firm agreement amongst experts as to whether it is preferable to have open types of freely ventilated natural convection housing or controlled-environment housing in hot climates. The author's preference is to use naturally ventilated housing with relatively light stocking densities wherever there are doubts about the reliability of the power supply, or the management skills are relatively unsophisticated. Buildings such as those shown in Figures 16.1 and 16.2 will give ideal conditions in most warm climates and there is a great facility for variation in the amount of ventilation and air movement by the use of controllable curtains at the front or sides of the building. This is generally essential as diurnal variations in temperature and air movement can be very great in tropical climates.

In nearly all circumstances it is desirable that the roof of the building is insulated to a high standard, equivalent to about 150 mm of glass fibre or 100 mm of expanded plastic. The outer claddings should be in light, heat-reflective materials.

The width of naturally ventilated houses should not exceed 13 m (40 ft) and the ridge height should be up to 4 m (13 ft) with a generous opening at the ridge up to 0.6 m (2 ft), suitably capped to prevent rain entry. A sharp-angled pitch to the roof will help ventilation to be effective. There should also be an overhang on the roof beyond the eaves of up to 1 m (3 ft) to give protection from the heat of the mid-day sun. The curtain at the front or side

Fig. 16.1 Span building for birds in hot climates.

Fig. 16.2 Monopitch building for birds in hot climates.

should extend over 70–80 per cent of the area and can, if desired, be controlled automatically by thermostats and motors with emergency 'fail-safe release' for high temperatures. Stocking rates for these types of buildings would be no more than about seven broilers per m^2 (15 kg body weight per m^2) or four or five layers or three or four breeders per m^2, depending on the size of the birds.

High air speeds are of great benefit to the birds and the attendant as they increase the heat loss by convection. Nevertheless, it must be stressed that these speeds should be higher than are normal in poultry houses and there is some danger that if the temperature goes above 41°C, which is the body temperature of the bird, high air speeds will *increase* the stress on the birds. Because of the importance of being able to increase the air movement whenever it is needed in naturally ventilated housing, it must be possible to open up as much as possible of the walls of the house without restriction. In addition it is advisable to incorporate the design ability to open up the sides 100 per cent in

very warm areas. Careful thought must also be given to the siting of naturally ventilated buildings so that the best use can be made of winds to flow
through the house when required.

Controlled-environment housing

This system is especially advocated for heavy weight broiler breeders or heavy
broilers which cannot stand very high temperatures because of their bulk and
therefore poorer heat-dissipating abilities. It is also widely favoured for
large cage laying houses where natural ventilation presents too many circulation difficulties. Stocking densities can be between 50 to 100 per cent more
than naturally ventilated housing and the principal features of controlled-
environment housing are as follows.

A high standard of thermal insulation is the first essential. The whole building should be insulated to a standard of 100 mm polyurethane or the equivalent in other materials, as chosen. Mechanical ventilation should be installed
to a maximum of approximately double that in temperate climates, and advice
given earlier in Chapter 7 on ventilation. While all the systems illustrated in
Chapter 7 can also be used in hot climates, there is a general preference for
positive pressure arrangements, as they enable a better control of air movement. Reliable electricity supplies and stand-by generators must be available.

It is noteworthy that building structures with a large thermal mass reduce
the diurnal variations in temperature and in this way lower the extremes of
environmental temperatures experienced by the birds. To put it more simply,
such buildings are slower to warm up in the day or to cool down at night. In
many parts of the world there are local materials that are ideally suited for
this purpose, for example, light-weight clay bricks or forms of aerated concrete. In buildings so constructed, the potentially large diurnal swings of temperature may also be further reduced by increasing the ventilation rate during
the night and thereby cooling the whole structure of the house and then reducing the ventilation from its maximum in the heat of the day so that the building materials have a better opportunity to remain cool. It would be especially
appropriate to use one of the water cooling methods described later during
the day to further assist the levelling out of temperature fluctuations. The temperature stresses that tend to kill poultry are caused largely by suddenly rising temperatures and/or humidity as the birds have had no ability to acclimatise
themselves and the method just described will be a significant help in preventing the most serious temperature stresses that kill the birds.

The main systems for keeping the birds cool use methods of evaporative
cooling, of which there are four principal forms. The simplest is the *pad or
filter system* in which the incoming air is drawn over a type of filter, often of

a cellulose material, which is kept soaked in water. Provision has to be made to protect the pad from excessive sand or dust, and recirculation and filtration of the water are usually also necessary.

A second system, also quite simple, is to use a series of *low pressure fogger nozzles* in the house, set up close to the ordinary fans or incoming air, to assist in the distribution of the mist. This system tends to become quickly clogged and easily leads to uneven conditions with the litter near the fogger becoming dangerously damp.

There are two superior arrangements. The first is by the use of a *spinning* disc to generate a spray of small droplets that are passed into a stream of air. The most popular of the disc coolers are horizontal free-standing units. However, a more recent development is the *ultra-high pressure mister* (Figure 16.3). In this case a pump is used to generate a high pressure in reinforced plastic distribution tubes fitted with special nozzles. The small droplet particles pass out into the house at about 100 m/s. The water supply must be carefully filtered and the pipes distributed in the house so that the incoming air will pick up the mist and help in the distribution.

The cooling systems described here are capable of lowering the ambient temperature in the house by a maximum of about 10°C (16°F) when relative humidity is down to around 30 per cent, but if the relative humidity is up to 50 per cent the effect will be nearer 6°C (10°F), with a rise in relative humidity to 80 per cent.

A much-used method where water is freely available is to trickle water over the roof of the house from perforated plastic pipes. The evaporation of the water will certainly have some beneficial effect and it also has the advantage

Fig. 16.3 Illustration of a high pressure misting (fogging) evaporation cooling system in a poultry house. (Courtesy of NRG Company, P.O. Box 306, Ardmore, PA 19003, USA.)

that this system does not raise the humidity of the air inside the house. It tends to be a method most favoured in those temperate climates where water is freely available and only occasionally are high temperatures met with. It is also cheap and easy to install a perforated plastic pipe along the ridge of the house and the occasional extravagance in water usage is a modest cost compared with the potential loss of birds suffering from heat stroke in large numbers. It is worthy of emphasis that high temperatures *per se* are by no means the only problem. High relative humidity, over about 70 per cent, is extremely serious and birds can perish in substantial numbers even at quite modestly high temperatures if they are given an abruptly severe heat stress. Without acclimatisation, heavy birds in particular are very susceptible to such conditions at high stocking densities.

Before poultry units are set up in potentially dangerous climates, the meteorological data should be carefully examined to establish whether the whole operation may be economically justified.

Feeding and watering in hot climates

Some birds will eat to their energy needs and as their energy requirement is obviously less in hot climates, it is essential to compensate for the inevitable reduction in food consumed. For example, with pullets being reared for laying or breeding, the protein content of the ration, which is usually at a level of 20 per cent to 4 weeks, then 15 per cent for 4 weeks and finally 12 per cent until the pullet is laying, should be amended to a level of 20 per cent, leaving it at this higher level until the pullets are housed for lay. It is also necessary to increase the vitamin and mineral content of the feed to the rearing bird and, as food consumption may be up to 20 per cent less at high temperatures, the vitamin and mineral levels should be increased to compensate by a similar margin of 20 per cent to give a safe, neither harmful nor wasteful, quantity. In addition, there should be an especially generous supply of drinkers; about 20 per cent more space should be provided than in temperate climates. Because of the danger of early dehydration, the first water provided for the young chick should have electrolytes and vitamins added to increase its attraction and value to the chick.

It is of benefit if the birds can actually dip their beaks in the water, thus drinkers with troughs are better than nipple systems. One of the ways in which birds keep cool is by losing heat from the comb and wattles and this ability will be greatly improved if they are kept moist. Only if there are fairly deep troughs can the birds thoroughly moisten these parts.

At high temperatures birds may consume twice, or exceptionally even three times as much water as at the normal range of ambient temperatures. Unless this water can be properly provided, there will not only be insufficient for the physiological functions of the bird but there may also be a serious reduction in feed consumption. For each kilogram of feed the bird may drink up to 3 kg of water. In addition, the cooler the water that can be provided, the better, and water storage facilities should therefore be protected from excessive radiation effects from the sun.

The food for all other ages and classes of birds should receive the same consideration, assuming about 20 per cent less consumption, and increasing the protein, mineral and vitamin percentages by an approximately pro rata amount.

In order to encourage food consumption in hot climates when controlled environment housing is used it is worthwhile giving the hours of darkness during the heat of the day and lighting the birds during the cooler night time. In fact not only will this encourage food consumption, it will also help to reduce the heat stress on the birds by encouraging them to rest during the day.

Some important additional points must be made. Deterioration in some of the essential micro-ingredients at high temperatures may readily take place and since transportation of feed ingredients over long distances and very uncertain storage conditions are almost inevitable, it is advised that if there is uncertainty about the quality, analyses should be carried out to check the position. Furthermore, under such uncertain conditions the growth of moulds producing pathogenic mycotoxins is more likely than in cool temperatures and it becomes essential to ensure the best feasible storage condition or to consider the possibility of incorporating an anti-mould agent in the food. In any event, an examination for mycotoxins in the food may be necessary.

Poultry diseases in hot climates

The health position tends to be worse in hot climates than in temperate areas. There are several reasons for this. First and foremost there is not the same tradition for hygiene in many such areas and yet paradoxically pathogenic microorganisms can often survive for a longer time in a warm environment, this being particularly true of some of the most devastating bacterial infections such as salmonella, pasteurella and clostridia. Several strains of these organisms also cause diseases that are communicable to man, such as food poisoning and gangrenous infections. Also, in hot climates there are greater infestations of the vectors that cause disease; biting insects, flies and mites may abound and these can be carriers and a reservoir of many diseases, especially those of viral origin. Usually there will also be considerable deficiencies in the immune protection chicks have derived from their parents so that they may receive serious challenges from disease-producing organisms as soon as they go into the house at day-old.

Provided these dangers are understood, proper measures can be taken to prevent their worst effects. In addition to the environmental and nutritional points already made, the following extra measures deserve emphasis.

- Maintain the cleanliness of the site at the highest standards, ensuring no accumulations of litter are left near the birds as the vectors of disease may live and thrive in these.
- Take the greatest care to keep visitors away unless they are fully protected by antiseptics and clean clothing.
- Apply a fully integrated programme of preventive vaccination which is tailored to local knowledge of the disease incidence.
- Protect the birds when necessary at times of stress with antibiotic medication for short controlled periods under veterinary direction.
- Exclude vermin and wild birds from the housing by suitable wire mesh over all ventilation and other open areas.
- Dispose of dead carcasses well away from the site or best of all by incineration.

It is as well to bear in mind that disease and environmental challenges will be much reduced if the birds are given more space than in cold and temperate areas.

17 Poultry Welfare and Alternative Systems

It has already been stressed in earlier sections of this book that there is considerable world-wide concern about the possible inhumanity involved in some of the modern poultry production systems. The objections have arisen for two principal reasons: the restriction on the movement of birds that such systems as the battery cage impose, and the barren nature of the birds' surroundings, with their whole lives spent squatting on a wire floor and being restricted by wire mesh or metal. Considerable investigation has been done and continues to be carried out in a scientific manner to try and establish the birds' mental and physiological reactions to environments such as the battery cage, and results show clearly the stresses caused by severe restrictions on movement and barren environments. The most satisfactory approach at present is perhaps epitomised in the codes of practice devised by the UK Farm Animal Welfare Council. This states that all farm animals should be provided with the following.

1. Comfort and shelter.
2. Freedom from thirst, hunger or malnutrition.
3. Freedom of movement.
4. Prevention or rapid diagnosis and treatment of vice, injury and disease.
5. The company of other animals, particularly of like kind.
6. The opportunity to display most normal patterns of behaviour.
7. Adequate lighting.
8. Flooring which neither harms nor causes undue strain.
9. The avoidance of unnecessary mutilation.
10. Emergency arrangements to cover fires and breakdowns.

A debate will doubtless continue for many years on the definition and interpretation of these clauses, but under modern intensive systems the principal difficulty is with item 6, the opportunity to display most normal patterns of behaviour. For chickens this could well be said, as many insist it does, that the bird must be able to stand up, sit down, turn round, flap its wings, have dust baths and lay its egg in a bedded nest.

Alternative systems for the management of laying poultry

The cage system of housing laying poultry is without doubt the most economical method of producing eggs. Furthermore, cage systems have regularly become more intensive by a steady increase in the number of tiers of cages in battery blocks. Arrangements with as many as eight tiers have been built. However, although the productivity and health of birds are better than other systems, there are serious welfare disadvantages in the cage system. Cages not only fail to provide the all-important welfare requirements of freedom of movement, freedom from fear, comfort and shelter, suitable flooring and freedom to display most normal patterns of behaviour, but also increase certain metabolic problems such as bone fragility.

Since cages for poultry were first criticised by animal welfare groups some 35 years ago there have been continuous endeavours to develop alternative systems that can provide a satisfactory level of welfare and also competitive productivity. However, these systems have incurred problems of poor productivity, increased disease incidence, intensive management, aggression and cannibalism. All such systems are more costly than cages as a method of producing eggs. An outline of some of these methods is given below.

The 'get-away' cage (Figure 17.1)

The very first welfare-orientated cage was produced about 20 years ago and had within it perches, nest boxes and 'dust baths'. There are a number of alternative arrangements of these. Such designs have found little following due to their expense and some management problems. However, they are being further developed, e.g. with time-monitored opening and closing of nests and sand baths.

The Elson tiered terrace (Figure 17.2)

A more recent system, developed by Dr Arnold Elson of the UK Agriculture and Development Advisory Service, is a tiered 'terrace' which aims to combine good control of the birds and 'high' technology of cages with the allowance of more freedom for the birds. Tiered sloping, wire mesh-floored terraces are interconnected by a 'stairwell' giving controlled access in the afternoon to a littered ground floor area.

Fig. 17.1 Get-away cage (Elson, 1976).

Fig. 17.2 Elson tiered terrace (ETT system).

Feed, water, nesting and perches are provided on each terrace, so that birds return to them at night via one-way gates. So far testing has shown that production can be good but cannibalism may be a problem.

The aviary system (Figures 17.3–17.5)

There are a number of aviary systems; these were the first of the multi-tiered alternatives to the cage which gave freedom of movement for birds within an intensive housing arrangement. The multi-tier arrangement approximates more closely to a bird's natural habitat. Temperature, ventilation and lighting are controlled and the vertical height of the house is made use of by allowing the

Fig. 17.3 Aviary at Gleadthorpe, England.

Fig. 17.4 Swiss aviary – 'Natura 280'.

Fig. 17.5 TWF aviary (The Netherlands).

birds to live at a number of different levels on slats, perches or wire floors. In addition there is always a littered area and nest boxes. The problems faced with this system are similar to those in the perchery arrangement described below.

The perchery system (Figure 17.6)

Although there are a number of alternative arrangements, the system consists essentially of a series of perches or slatted platforms, usually on an A-frame over a wire floor, which allows the droppings to fall either into a deep pit or on to a belt from which they can then be scraped away. Such systems allow a high density of stocking but with both the aviary and perchery systems there may be feather pecking, cannibalism, floor and broken eggs and high disease incidence. Figure 17.6 shows an arrangement of this type of system pioneered by Dr Michie in Scotland.

Fig. 17.6 Michie perchery (Scotland).

Sloping wire floors (Pennsylvania systems)

A variety of sloping wire-floor systems has been developed from the original Pennsylvania system where the birds were confined to a sloping wire floor on which they lived their entire life and also laid their eggs. Modern developments may include nest boxes, perches and sanded scratching areas. The customary behavioural problems occur, cannibalism, feather pecking and egg-eating. One such system is that produced by Dr Hans Kier (Figure 17.7) and is currently being used in Denmark.

Fig. 17.7 Plan and cross-section of the Hans Kier system (Denmark).

Tiered developments of the original sloping wire floors

These use several levels of floors incorporating automatic belt collection of manure, and perches and littered floors for scratching and dust bathing. These are often high-density systems with birds housed at 20 birds per square metre and could show considerable promise if the behavioural problems in high stocking rates can be overcome.

Deep litter

The deep-litter system was first developed in its modern form some 50 years ago and, with improvements, is generally used for breeders. The house has built-up litter of wood shavings or chopped straw, a controlled environment, automatic feeding and drinking, nest boxes that may have automatic egg collection, and in many cases an area of perches over a droppings pit. The

Ventilating open ridge

6 ft
(1·8 m)

Wire front covered with polythene panels in winter

Solid base

FRONT ELEVATION

Ventilator

Slate

Ventilated gable and end walls

6 ft
(1·8 m)

Solid base part of walls

20 ft (6 m)

END ELEVATION

Ventilation

Hanging feeder or drinker

Nest boxes

6 ft
(1·8 m)

Perch units

Litter 1 ft deep
(50 cms)

CROSS SECTION

20 ft (8 m)

Nest boxes
(1 per 4 birds)

Tubular drinkers

20 ft
(6 m)

Movable perch units

Tubular feeders

Divided sections
30 ft (9 m) x 20 ft (8 m)
to take 200 birds

Access from front for cleaning

PLAN OF COVERED STRAW YARD

Fig. 17.8 Plans of covered straw yard.

system is satisfactory provided stocking density is not excessive. It is an expensive system to erect and to manage and for these reasons is not currently used very much for commercial egg layers.

Covered straw yard (barn system) (Figure 17.8)

Birds are kept in a simple covered yard which is deeply strawed. Ventilation is by natural air flow and lighting likewise, supplemented only by artificial lighting when necessary. The straw litter is kept at a depth of about 500 mm and is constantly topped up to keep it to this depth at least. Food and water supply is automatic, egg production is good but feed consumption may increase due to absence of environmental control. Birds may roost on perches in a separate insulated area. The birds should not be stocked above four birds per square metre and should be kept in groups of not more than 200–300. Vices may develop if the birds are overstocked. The system is easy to run, especially if units are of modest size, and the system has had a following for years.

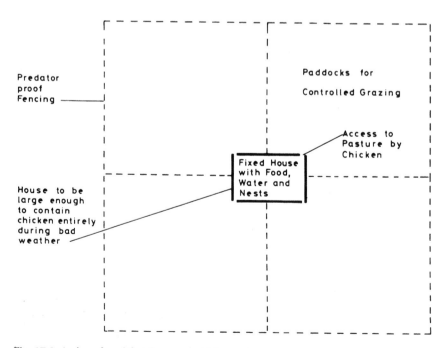

Fig. 17.9 A plan of modified free-range chicken unit.

Table 17.1 Estimates of egg production costs in different poultry systems

System	Space	Cost
Laying cage	450 cm^2/bird	100
Laying cage	560 cm^2/bird	105
Laying cage	750 cm^2/bird	115
Laying cage	450 cm^2/bird + perch	100
Laying cage	450 cm^2/bird + perch and nest	102
Get-away cage and 2-tier aviary	10–12 birds/m^2	110 / 115
Aviary and perchery and multi-tier housing	20 birds/m^2	108
Deep litter	7–10 birds/m^2	118
Straw yard	3 birds/m^2	130
Free range	1000 birds/hectare	150

Indices are based on the percentage over laying cages stocked at 450 cm^2/bird.

Free range (Figure 17.9)

This is a system where birds are given free access to pasture and for egg-laying poultry they must not be stocked above 1000 birds per hectare. The house itself is virtually the same as deep-litter or perchery housing.

The system is only economic because the return on 'free-range' eggs is better than from 'barn' eggs, which are those from the alternative systems. The system can run into problems from cannibalism, floor eggs and dirty eggs. Food consumption and labour demands are high. Disease can be a problem if the land is overused. Bad weather and predators may cause difficulties. The highest standards of stockmanship are essential. Well-designed thermally insulated portable free-range houses are now available.

Semi-intensive systems

This is the traditional domestic poultry keeper's method, with a small fixed timber house leading to one or more open runs. The arrangement is only satisfactory for small groups of birds as it has serious environmental, labour, productivity, health and hygienic disadvantages.

Free-range table chicken

An increasing number of table chicken are now produced under free range conditions. There are a number of features that are fundamentally different from the intensive broiler bird. Instead of a fast growing broiler strain, the real free-range table bird is red feathered, slower growing and maturing so that it takes nearly twice as long to reach a similar weight as a broiler. After the first 2–3 weeks of life brooded on straw or wood shavings, the birds are given free access to pasture. The diet is generally largely cereal, with the sufficient addition of vegetable protein, vitamins and minerals, but no animal protein is added nor are growth promoters given, and the protein content and energy levels are several percentage points below broiler diets.

It is claimed that with the extra time taken to mature, the flavour is improved and indeed a bird is offered with a more traditional chicken flavour. It also has much less fat than the broiler bird.

Conclusions

It is not easy to foresee clearly where the welfare controversy is going to lead. Research and investigation may eventually provide a scientific answer but in many ways the moral issue has tended to make the running and will probably overrule the scientific evidence. Our legislators, moved by public demand, are now almost certain to consider the keeping of layers in multi-bird cages unacceptable, in which case it is good to know that there are a number of alternative arrangements that can be used to provide eggs of good quality at modest extra cost, other than those laid by the cage bird.

However, if the alternative systems to battery cages are to be successful in all respects, including welfare, the poultryman must be aware of the skills required. Some of the most popular trends affecting the evolution of the modern poultry industry will be abruptly halted or reversed and these must be considered in a practical manner.

Over several generations commercial egg layers have been expertly bred for their efficiency under cage conditions and there will have to be changes in genetic selection techniques if the ideal strains for future needs are to be produced.

Diseases are likely to be on the increase unless great care is taken. The birds can more readily get infested with parasites and other agents of disease in most alternative systems unless the litter is kept in a dry and friable state and only modest stocking rates are allowed. There will also be a revived risk of vices occurring, such as feather pecking and cannibalism. There is unlikely to be any desire to trim the beaks of birds and the prevention of vices will depend entirely on skilled management.

Cages with sloping wire bases almost certainly ensure that eggs are clean with no need for effort on the part of the attendant, but it can be very different with floor systems. If all the birds use the nest boxes provided and these are kept clean there is no problem but, quite unpredictably, there may be a tendency for some or even many birds to lay their eggs on the floor. This has many dangers. The eggs will probably be dirty and at worst could be a danger to health. Some eggs may get broken accidentally and this may set in train 'egg-eating' which can cause a serious loss of eggs. A great deal of investigation is currently being undertaken into the behaviour of laying birds in an endeavour to ensure that nests are correctly designed and sited to encourage birds to use them exclusively, but there are so many differences in the behaviour of various strains of birds that it is too much to expect total success.

It must be repeated that the final results depend on management. Just as the cage system has been the main factor that has encouraged the growth of the mammoth egg-laying units, so may the development of alternative systems see a change to smaller groups of birds in smaller buildings and on smaller poultry units. Many may applaud such a development, which will not only be an aid to good management but may also make better use of the resources of the land. It is much more likely that the smaller unit will utilise locally produced feedstuffs and the litter at the end of the crop will be of great value to the land. In large intensive units, on the other hand, the poultry feed may have to be hauled a great distance and the manure at the end of a crop is a liability. If we can also see the removal of some of the hazards inherent in systems that are totally dependent on mechanical environmental control and feeding, there can be improved management since time is spent on inspection of and caring for the birds rather than on the repair of the machinery.

Poultry husbandry is an exciting subject and nothing stays the same for long. At the moment we are at one of the most crucial and interesting stages in its development, where welfare concerns are having a profound influence on the direction in which poultry systems are moving. Readers are referred to the Ministry of Agriculture's Codes of Recommendations for Poultry Welfare produced in the United Kingdom together with reports on poultry welfare published by the Farm Animal Welfare Council.

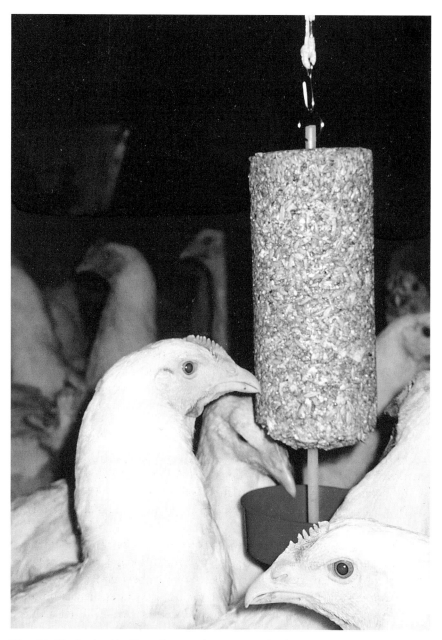

Plate 22 The 'peck-a-block' – a device to hang in a poultry house to provide a useful diversion for birds on floor systems. It is based on cereal suitably compressed to provide a lengthy activity.

18 Organic Poultry Production

The public is increasingly eager to seek food products which are produced under 'natural' conditions; not just free range but organic. Such is the demand for these in the UK that some 70 per cent of organic products sold here are imported. Yet the criteria for producing organic poultry and eggs are clearly laid down, and can form a profitable enterprise.

Organic food production in general is defined by European Union law and is based on the following principles:

- Building soil fertility.
- Minimal use of non-renewable resources (no chemicals).
- Minimal pollution and damage to the environment.
- Working with, not against, natural systems.
- Respect for animal welfare.
- Minimal processing or additives.

Organic farming is governed by an EU regulation No. 2092/91 (as amended). At the request of the Ministry of Agriculture, Fisheries and Food, an independent third party organisation was set up by 'Food from Britain' known as the United Kingdom Register of Organic Food Standards (UKROFS).

UKROFS is empowered to set production standards for and establish a register of approved producers of organic foodstuffs. It is governed by a board under an independent chairman, composed of members with a wide range of interests in organic foodstuffs, including producers, processors, distributors, consumers and enforcement authorities. The Board and its Chairman are appointed by Agricultural Ministers and this ensures that no one interest predominates. The Board of UKROFS was established to be the UK certifying authority for organic foods and has since become the control authority under the EU regulation for organic production already referred to. The Board is charged with the following tasks:

1. To set production standards for organic produce tied to a UK organic symbol.
2. To consider applications from organic sector bodies to check that their proposed standards are at least equivalent to the standard set under (1) and are supported by adequate inspection arrangements.
3. To consider applications from individual producers of organic food not linked to a recognised body, to ensure that their standards conform to the standards under (1) and are supported by adequate inspection arrangements.
4. To establish a register of individual organic producers whereby registration provides a right to use the symbol.

**UKROFS STANDARDS
FOR ORGANIC FOOD PRODUCTION**

Fig. 18.1 Logos to be found on organically produced poultry products.

In the ensuing paragraphs the standards required by UKROFS and the Soil Association are summarised to give any intending producer a general statement of those details that are necessary if it is intended to go into organic production. General standards applying to all poultry are as follows.

While in general all livestock intended for meat production must be born and live their entire lives on an organic unit, poultry are an exception in that they may be brought in from conventional systems at 1 day old. Poultry for egg production may be brought in up to 16 weeks of age and must undergo a conversion period of 6 weeks during which time they must be managed in accordance with organic standards before the eggs are sold under an organic designation.

An objective of organic agriculture is to sustain animals in good health by the adoption of effective management practices, including high standards for animal welfare, appropriate diets, good stockmanship and preventing conditions where the use of remedial treatments, particularly chemotherapy, becomes necessary. All livestock must be handled, housed and transported under conditions which reflect proper care and concern for their welfare at all times and which comply at least with the requirements of all relevant legislation and MAFF codes of recommendations for animal welfare. The breeds and strains of livestock selected must be suitable for raising under local conditions under an organic regime. The use of artificial insemination in the breeding programme (e.g. turkeys) is permitted. Cockerels may be brought in for breeding purposes and no conversion period is required.

Animal health and welfare in organic systems

Special care is required in nurturing and encouraging positive health and vitality, ensuring the proper control of disease and the encouragement of 'positive animal welfare' (PAW). The term PAW means satisfying the birds' needs in a way that provides for their behavioural requirements, not just negatively avoiding cruelty.

Preventive chemotherapy can only be used to deal with specifically identified diseases or as part of an agreed conversion or disease reduction plan. Such a plan must be agreed between the farmer and a nominated veterinary surgeon and after conversion to develop and operate an organic livestock system that conforms to UKROFS standards. This arrangement must ensure the development of a pattern of health building and disease control measures appropriate to the particular circumstances of the individual farm. Homeopathy may form part of the agreed plan, where it is appropriate. The plan should ensure proper animal welfare at all times but should allow for the evolution of a farming system less dependent on chemotherapy.

Certain animal health control practices are allowed on a routine basis, such as anthelminthics for worms by agreement with the nominated veterinary surgeon and to be accompanied by husbandry practices designed to reduce or where possible eliminate the presence of unacceptable worm infestation. Vaccination is also permitted where there is a known disease risk, and also the use of antibiotics and other conventional medication to treat disease under the advice of the nominated veterinary surgeon, where effective alternative treatments are not available and where they are considered to be the best method of reducing suffering, saving life or restoring an animal to health. No 'growth promoters' are allowed. All veterinary medicines must be used in accordance with their UK product licence or as directed by the prescribing veterinarian. Withdrawal times between the end of the treatment and using the product from the animal when medicines in the following classification are used should be:

1. At least double that defined by the product licence and not less than 14 days in the case of:
   (a) controlled drugs
   (b) prescription-only medicines
   (c) pharmacist-only medicines
   (d) veterinary products appearing on the Merchant's list.
2. As defined by the product licence or by the prescribing veterinarian in the case of veterinary products appearing on the general sale list.

Welfare and housing

Housing and management must be appropriate to the behavioural needs of the birds. All stock must have sufficient room to stand naturally, lie down easily, turn round, groom themselves, assume all natural postures and make all natural movements such as stretching and wing flapping and to walk about freely at least in accordance with MAFF Codes of Practice for poultry welfare.

All houses should be well bedded with straw or other appropriate material. Up to 25 per cent of the floor can be slatted. Birds must not be subjected to any surgical or chemical interference that is not designed to improve the birds own health or well-being.

Poultry diets

All poultry should be planned to provide 100 per cent of the diet from feedstuffs produced to UKROFS standards. However, in cases where this is not immediately possible, at least 50 per cent of the dry matter in the diet must

Table 18.1 Brought-in approved feedstuffs from non-organic sources fed according to the following daily allowances (kg DM)

Bird type	Total daily DMS	Daily non-organic allowance
Layers	0.118	0.024
Table birds	0.077	0.015
Turkeys	0.138	0.027
Geese	0.150	0.030
Ducks	0.150	0.030

come from feedstuffs produced to UKROFS standards. The balance of the specified minimum organic part of the diet, 70 per cent, may come from registered holdings which are in the process of conversion to organic production providing the holding has been inspected, the production plan has been accepted by an approved body and after a conversion period of at least 12 months before harvest has been complied with. The balance may be brought in from other sources providing the sources are known to the producer and are registered with an approved body.

The diets must be balanced, of good quality, and should not have levels of protein and energy or other additions associated with intensive production. Materials that have been subjected to solvent extraction are prohibited.

Good management

All poultry production systems must be planned to allow the birds to have continuous and easy daytime access to open-air runs, except in adverse weather conditions. The land to which the birds have access must be adequately covered with properly managed and suitable vegetation. In the case of egg production, where a conventional unit is run in conjunction with the organic unit, birds of the same species may not be kept unless the resulting egg production is identifiable by colour.

Where set stocking is practised, stocking rates should not exceed 250 birds/acre. Pasture should be rested for 1 year in three where set stocking is practised. Permanent housing of poultry is prohibited. Colony sizes recommended are: not more than 100 laying birds per housing group or 200 for meat birds, but permitted are up to 500 per housing group. For layers, artificial lighting must not prolong the day length beyond 16 hours. Recommended housing spaces for layers are: 15 kg live weight per square metre of floor area, 20 cm perch space per bird and one nest space for five birds.

For layers the following are permitted: fixed houses with slatted floors for collection area for droppings and/or solid floors with litter. Houses moved twice per week may have slatted floors with no droppings boards. Also permitted is housing designed for a maximum of 25 kg of birds per square metre of floor area, 15 cm of perch space per bird and one nest box per eight birds.

Fattening birds

Recommended are 18 kg of birds per square metre of floor area, 75 per cent of floor area littered, and 25 per cent of the area as a raised stalled or weld-mesh roosting area with enclosed droppings collection area below, but permitted is housing designed for a maximum of 25 kg live weight, mature birds or 12 birds per square metre, which is approximately one bird per square foot. No other floor arrangements or stocking densities are permitted and no beak trimming is allowed.

Conclusions

It is clear that rearing birds to comply with organic standards is an exacting commitment. However, products command a much better return and with demand increasing and home production being quite insufficient, it is well worth consideration, especially as a means of poultry farming that is suited to the smaller operator as part of a less specialised livestock farm. It is necessary that methods of poultry farming change in line with the public's demands and legislative requirements.

Further Reading

1. General management

Anon. (1989) *Poultry Serviceman's Manual.* Rahway, NJ: Merck, Sharpe & Dohme.

Anon. (1999) *Poultry and Eggs.* London: Poultry World Technical Publications.

Appleby, M.C., Hughes, D.O. and Elson, H.A. (1992) *Poultry Production.* Wallingford: CABI.

Bartleff, T. (1990) *Ducks and Geese: A Guide to Management.* Swindon: Crowood Press.

Cole, D.J.A. and Brander, G.C. (1986) *Bioindustrial Ecosystems.* Amsterdam: Elsevier.

Ducks and Geese (1983) Bulletin No. 70, Ministry of Agriculture, Fisheries and Food (MAFF). London: HMSO.

Ewbank, R., Molslien, K. and Hart, C.B. (1999) *Management and Welfare of Farm Animals* (4th edn). Potters Bar: Universities Federation for Animal Welfare.

Gleadthorpe Experimental Husbandry Farm Reports (1974 onwards), MAFF. London: HMSO.

Lampkin, N. (1998) *Organic Farming.* Ipswich: Farming Press.

Robbins, G.E.S. (1989) *Quail, Their Breeding and Management.* Reading: World Pheasant Association.

Robbins, G.E.S. (1990) *Introduction to Quail in Captivity.* Reading: World Pheasant Association.

Thompson, M.A. (1978) *The Organic Poultryman.* Bridport, Dorset: Matthew A. Thompson.

Whittle, T. (1998) *A Triumph of Science.* London. Poultry World.

World Poultry Science Journals published by The World's Poultry Science Association. Published regularly with invaluable articles and reviews.

2. Breeding, hatching and welfare

Baxter, S.H., Baxter, M.R. and MacCormack, J.A.O. (1983) *Farm Animal Housing and Welfare.* The Hague: Nijhoff.

Jones, D.R. and Hodgetts, B. (1987) *Incubation and Hatchery Practice.* Bulletin No. 148, MAFF. London: HMSO.

Koene, P. and Blokhuis, H.J. (1997) *Proceedings of Fifth European Symposium on Poultry Welfare.*

Lake, P.E. and Stewart, J.M. (1978) *Artificial Insemination in Poultry.* Bulletin No. 213, MAFF. London: HMSO.

Romanoff, A.L. (1960) *The Avian Embryo.* New York: Macmillan.

Romanoff, A.L. and Romanoff, A.J. (1949) *The Avian Egg.* New York: John Wiley.

Sainsbury, D. (1988) *Farm Animal Welfare.* Oxford: Blackwell Scientific.

Savory, C.J. and Hughes, B.O. (1993) Fourth European Symposium on Poultry Welfare. Potters Bar: Universities Federation for Animal Welfare.

3. Nutrition

Agricultural Research Council (1975) *Nutrient Requirements of Farm Livestock – Poultry (1975).* London: Agricultural Research Council.

Ewing, W.R. (1983) *Poultry Nutrition.* Pasadena: The Roy Ewing Co.

Leeson, S. and Summers, J.D. (1991) *Commercial Poultry Nutrition.* Ontario: University Books.

McDonald, P., Edwards, R.A. and Greenhalgh, J.F.D. (1988) *Animal Nutrition* (4th edn). Harlow: Longman.

4. Environment and housing

Appleby, M.C. and Hughes, B.O. (1991) Welfare of Laying Hens. *World Poultry Science Journal,* 47(2): 109–128.

Charles, D.R. and Spencer, P.G. (1976) *The Climatic Environment of Poultry Houses,* Bulletin No. 212, MAFF. London: HMSO.

Esmay, M.L. (1979) *Principles of Animal Environment.* Westport, CT: AVI Publishing.

International Office of Epizootics (1991) *Animals, Pathogens and the Environment – A Review.* Paris: International Office of Epizootics.

Sainsbury, D. and Sainsbury, P. (1988) *Livestock Health and Housing.* London: Ballière Tindall.

Thear, K. (1997) *Free Range Poultry.* Ipswich: Farming Press Books.

Wathes, C.M. and Charles, D.R. (1944) *Livestock Housing.* Wallingford: CABI.

Woolcock, J.B. (1991) *Microbiology of Animals and Animal Products.* World Animal Science, A6. Amsterdam: Elsevier.

5. Poultry health

Altmaun, B., Clubb, S., Dorresheim, G. and Queensberry, K. (1997) *Avian Medicine and Surgery.* Philadelphia, PA: W.B. Saunders.

Curtis, P. (1990) *Poultry and Game Bird Diseases.* Liverpool: Liverpool University Press.

Gordon, R.F. and Freeman, B.M. (1971) *Poultry Diseases and World Economy.* BEMB Symposium No 7. Edinburgh: Longman.

Hofstad, M.A. *et al.* (1986) *Diseases of Poultry* (7th edn). Ames, IA: Iowa State University Press.

Jordan, F.T.W. ed. (1990) *Poultry Diseases* (3rd edn). London: Ballière Tindall.

Merck & Co. (1991) *Merck Veterinary Manual* (7th edn). Rahway, NJ: Merck & Co.

Pattison, M. (1993). *The Health of Poultry.* London: Longman.

Index